"Great read! Here is a ten-year walk down the path of a scary Trisomy birth that leads us to the 'pure, unadulterated joy these children can bring.'"
— John Wells, Board Member of L'Arche London, Ontario; Husband and Father

"This story turns broken into whole, tragedy into joy, and optimism into hope. Nancy is an inspiration for all parents struggling with a child with challenges."
— Debby Elnatan, Inventor of Upsee, a children's walking device, and Mom

"Nancy, it's a wonder when someone does what you do, in *Up, Not Down Syndrome*—namely, puts a searchlight into the nooks and crannies of one's own experience to shine the light of day on our shared humanity. And you offer many little 'epiphanies' along the way, beginning on the first page of Chapter 1, where you write, 'But we cannot know life's later lessons in the moment. We can only be where we are.' Thank you for this."
— Brenda Dixon-Gottschild, Ph.D., Author, Lecturer, Consultant, Teacher, Performer, and Prof. Emerita, Dance Studies, Temple University

"Nancy's story shines a powerful light on the murky waters of parenting and family dynamics. A required read for any parent navigating the occasionally cloudy and sometimes dark waters of parenthood and family. You will laugh, cry, and love. Enjoy the ride. I'm humbled by this love story."
— Beth Nordman, Giving Bean Coffee

"Nancy Schwartz's *Up, Not Down Syndrome* reverberates with such love and care, not just for her son Alex, but for all the friends, family, medical professionals, educators, support staff, physical therapists, and numerous others with whom she has created community. This book shows how a child and a family can impact the world in a powerful, hope-filled way. I felt privileged to read this story."
— Elizabeth Castiglione, Artist and Mother

"Having a child with Down syndrome has enriched my life in the best possible way by introducing me to an amazing community filled with parents passionate about helping their children grow and learn to the best of their abilities. Through CHOP Buddy Walk, I have come to know Nancy and her son, Alex. Nancy's resolve to ensure that Alex and his brothers thrive has influenced me to reach further for my own son and his siblings and become a Down syndrome advocate. I'm so thankful that Nancy put pen to paper to document her personal experiences in *Up, Not Down Syndrome*. In this book, Nancy shares personal testimony that can be helpful to a wide range of audiences—from those who can benefit from understanding the wide range of emotions that parents of children with disabilities can face to those who can benefit from the ways Nancy is able to see and develop Alex's abilities; there are lessons in this book that can help any and every reader. The three components of each chapter, the storytelling, the Lessons Alex Taught Me, and Alex's unique perspective combine to help the reader understand that Alex's life has tremendous value and potential. I will recommend this book to families who have recently received a medical diagnosis, to extended families within our Down syndrome community, to teachers and support staff and to students. Thank you, Nancy, for sharing your story with the world!"
— Danielle Thompson, Mom to Porter, Penny, and Paxton, Wife, and CPA

"The truth and beauty of Nancy Schwartz's words tell an ongoing story of love, learning, and the power of acceptance. All can learn from this family's boundless hope and from their source of joy and strength: Alex."
— April Beard, Music Educator and Cellist

"With indomitable tenderness, *Up, Not Down Syndrome* reveals the unexpected wonder of raising a son with Downs syndrome. Get ready for a brilliant love."
— Deidre Schena, Historian and Mother

"This is a wonderful book to remind you that the joy of love is possible in unexpected places when you open your heart to it."
— Barbara Taylor Bowman,
Irving B. Harris Professor of Child Development

"This book is an inspiration and a challenge, calling each of us to look at the ways in which we need to expand our hearts and minds. Reading about Alex, I felt an inner tug to move beyond my preconceived notions and limiting beliefs. This isn't simply a story about a mother's love for her son. It's a call-to-action. Each and every one of us can expand to greater love if only we look at the upside of the downs in our lives."
— Daralyse Lyons, Author, Actress, Speaker, Coach, and Yogi

"Once in a great while, there is a book that speaks directly to your heart. It uplifts you and pulls you in with a compelling story and a message that changes how you think. In *Up, Not Down Syndrome*, Nancy Schwartz shares her real-life story of giving birth to Alex, her son whose challenges and struggles catapulted her and her family into a whole new world and a whole new perspective on life. She shares her inner struggles, the real life drama of what happened, and her family's breathtaking victories. It's a story of learning to see the good, of gratitude, and growth. It's a must-read for people of all ages with its universal message of hope and light and love."
— Susie Garber, Educator, Mother, Grandmother, Reporter, Speaker, and Author

"This book is a lifeline to families who need support and encouragement. Nancy's soul-bearing story is inspirational, informative, and invaluable."
— Jackie Bratsis, Educator and Mother

"This book is for anyone wanting to know what it's like to raise a child with Down syndrome. In her memoir, Nancy Schwartz shares the initial fears that ultimately give way to celebrations, and lessons learned from her son, Alex. It is a moving and deeply insightful book that will open one's eyes to the joys of raising a child with Down syndrome."
— Jessica Wells, Quality Assurance Engineer and Teacher

"*Up, Not Down Syndrome* is an inspiring read. Nancy Schwartz will take you with her on her journey, touch your heart, and leave you full of more hope, love, and appreciation for life. Read it now!"
— Lisa Kohn, Speaker, Leadership Expert, and Author of the Best-Selling Memoir *to the moon and back*

"*Up, Not Down Syndrome* will challenge your notion that raising a differently-abled child is any sort of hardship. Instead, it is the greatest blessing bestowed upon us; we are not worthy. This book is a giant fist reaching into your chest, squishing your heart, changing everything you believed about parenting someone special. No nonsense storytelling but with Nancy's beautifully sculpted soul gleaming through each page. Be prepared to meet and fall in love with Alex and his posse, even if you spill tears on each page."
— Paige Figi, Adventurer, Executive Director of Coalition for Access Now, Mom to Charlotte, Chase, and Maxwell, Charlotte's Web CBD

"A moving and wise story of how a family navigates through hope, loss, learning, and most of all, love."
— Rabbi David Wolpe, Author of *David: The Divided Heart*

"I have been amazed at Nancy's advocacy for Alex and those like him. Through this book and by example, Nancy and her family are teaching us the gifts of the challenge. 'People will treat him the way I treat him,' is the quote I can hear her say over and over. Nancy so honestly shares her fear, shame, and anger that happened soon after Alex was born and how it transformed into acceptance, love, joy, and growth. *Up, Not Down Syndrome* will serve as a life raft for anyone in a similar situation because it teaches the rest of us about kindness and inclusivity. Beautifully, beautifully written."
— Jessica Lowenadler Sontag, Kitchen Coach, Wife, and Mom to Jonas, Mia, and Anders

"The story of Alex and his family is an important one to share! Nancy Schwartz is a fierce advocate and mother whose passion and love sound a call for the inclusive society we need."
— David Bradley, Theater Producer and Director of *A Fierce Kind of Love*, Produced by Temple University's Institute on Disabilities

"Raising a child is an act of faith. Raising a child with a disability requires a fierce kind of love. Nancy Schwartz invites us to share her unique journey of faith, love, and belonging. *Up, Not Down Syndrome* is more than the story of a family. It is a reflection on community, deepening our understanding of what it means to be truly human."
—Lisa Sonneborn, Director, Media Arts & Culture, Institute on Disabilities, Temple University

"'How can I love an imperfect child?' author Nancy Schwartz asks in her compulsively readable and heartwarming new book, *Up, Not Down Syndrome: Uplifting Lessons Learned from Raising a Son with Trisomy 21*. Through the pages of the book, Nancy learns that her new baby boy, Alex, will teach her how to love him and also how to embrace her new life in many happy and surprising ways. This is the story of one woman and one family embracing the challenges of raising a child with Trisomy 21 and finding that the daily battle of meeting those challenges results in a deepening bond and richer understanding of what it means to be human. Schwartz shows throughout the book that she is a learner and she effectively shows readers how committing to learning *about* her child and *from* her child made all the difference. Along the way, she learns that Alex is a great teacher, but also a great learner himself. This is a joyful book about one woman's and one family's heroic journey and one little boy's capacity to teach others lessons in life and love."
— Russ Walsh, Rider University, Author of *A Parent's Guide to Public Education in the 21st Century*

"A beautiful, honest account of not just accepting—but embracing—the unknown. Nancy shows us the blessing of an unexpected gift and the enormity of love."
— Sara Byala, PhD

Up, Not Down Syndrome

**Uplifting Lessons Learned
From Raising a Son With
Trisomy 21**

Nancy M. Schwartz

Modern History Press

Up, Not Down Syndrome: Uplifting Lessons Learned From Raising a
Son With Trisomy 21

Library of Congress Cataloging-in-Publication Data
Names: Schwartz, Nancy M., 1968- author.
Title: Up, not down syndrome : uplifting lessons learned from raising a son
  with Trisomy 21 / Nancy M. Schwartz.
Description: Ann Arbor, MI : Modern History Press, [2019] | Includes
  bibliographical references and index. | Summary: "When Alex is born with
  Down Syndrome (Trisomy 21) the author and her family decide to take
  care of him at home against the advice of doctors. The resulting life-
  lessons have taught the author that the happiness and joy that Alex
  brings is more than worth the struggle of parenting"-- Provided by
publisher.
Identifiers: LCCN 2019017596 (print) | LCCN 2019980364 (ebook) | ISBN
  9781615994632 (hardcover) | ISBN 9781615994625 (paperback) | ISBN
  9781615994649 (ebook)
Subjects: LCSH: Schwartz, Nancy M., 1968---Family. | Mothers of children
  with Down syndrome--United States--Biography. | Down
  syndrome--Patients--Care--United States--Biography. | Mothers and
  sons--United States--Biography.
Classification: LCC RJ506.D68 S337 2019   (print) | LCC RJ506.D68
(ebook) |
  DDC 618.92/8588420092 [B]--dc23
LC record available at https://lccn.loc.gov/2019017596
LC ebook record available at https://lccn.loc.gov/2019980364

Published by
Modern History Press
5145 Pontiac Trail
Ann Arbor, MI 48105

www.ModernHistoryPress.com
info@ModernHistoryPress.com

Tollfree 888-761-6268
FAX 734-663-6861

Cover design: Doug West / ZAQ Designs
Photo editing: Dylan Ball
Photo credits: Ellen Glazier Schwartz

For Josh, Sam, and Alex

"Do what makes your heart happy."
                                    Gina Cutlip Grandy

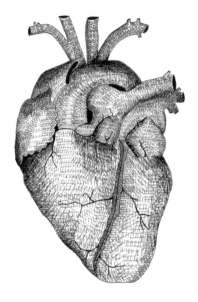

Human heart, drawing by Josh Schwartz

Contents

Introduction: The Story of Alex's Birth

Soon after our second son, Sam, was born, my husband, Michael, lost his job. My earnings had already been cut in half because I was on maternity leave from my teaching position, so our family endured a full year with no second income. But, as they do, things turned around.

Michael got a new job. I went back to school teaching English Language Learning (ELL). Sam, and his older brother, Josh, were happily developing into wonderful young boys.

Both Sam and Josh's teachers regularly regaled Michael and me with stories about how our boys helped their fellow classmates. When I went to pick up the boys at school, other parents would stop me to say what incredible, kind, sweet, amazing, fine, young men I was raising. And that was before our family was hit with what turned out to be the best of all possible disasters when our third son, Alex, was born.

Josh would be the one to say a last goodbye to Pop Pop when he passed on before the service at Goldstein's, in Bucks County, Pennsylvania. (Pop Pop is what the boys called their grandfather, Michael's father.) Josh is fearless. At age fourteen, Josh took the train to the city with friends. I was worried, but I needn't have been. Everything went well. Josh has always been advanced beyond his years. Responsible and fun.

I will never forget how Sam gave his stuffed bear, named Bear, to Alex. Bear stayed with Sam through his Pop Pop's passing, Alex's birth, and more. It has a majestic quality of love sewn in from a dime store on Long Beach Island. The day Sam gave Bear to Alex, I cried. I cried at his generosity, but also at the awareness that Sam was growing up.

I love Alex, Josh, and Sam more than anyone. I want them all to be healthy and happy. Luckily, Josh and Sam are continuing to flourish. They have remained pillars of hope and strength, unobtrusive and easy to please. There are billions of examples of how extraordinary both Sam and Josh are. When I think about all they will be, it fills me with a pride that does not end. When I see Sam walk his friend, Kayla, to the door, I think what a gorgeous and polite young man he is. My middle child balances the demands of playing on two soccer teams. As a high school student, he was on the varsity school soccer team for Upper Merion as well as the Prussians soccer club team. He played for Diamond baseball, and the Upper Merion High School baseball team. A gifted athlete, he also maintained uninterrupted honor roll status while taking a rigorous curriculum of honors classes. Josh is a beautiful young man. He has balanced running on the school's track team, working at the childcare center at the Lifetime gym three times a week, and getting honors in all his classes, including his advanced placement level courses. Josh's positive outlook is infectious. Both my older boys (young men, now, although I still see them as my boys) astound me with their love for Alex, and their ability to incorporate him into their busy lives.

When Michael and I found out we were expecting, for the *third* time, we were a mixture of overjoyed and freaked out. How would we continue to dig out from the year he hadn't worked? How would we support a new baby along with our two existing boys?

Sure, by then, Sam and Josh were five and six, and Michael had been back to work for awhile, but the impact of more than three-hundred-sixty-five unemployed days had taken their toll, as evidenced by our high credit card and low checking account balances. Also, I was forty. I thought I was done with middle-of-the-night feedings and diaper changes. I had a fulltime job as a teacher. My to-do list was never-ending. Yet, there was also an upsurge of excitement.

I love being a mother. Josh and Sam had given more shape and substance to my life than I could have ever imagined. Now, Michael and I would have a third.

The news that my third baby would be a boy could not have been more comforting.

You know what you're doing, I reassured myself. *You have done this twice before.*

It wasn't long before fear was eclipsed by a sense of unlimited possibilities.

What would my third son's personality be? Would he be sensitive and kind, like Josh? A true egalitarian, like Sam?

I couldn't wait to meet him. Evidently, he felt the same.

Near the end of my pregnancy, I went to a routine doctor's visit and was told I would not be going home.

Dr. Diamond pinched the bridge of his nose and closed his eyes. "Let's have you have this baby tonight," he said.

I knew something wasn't right. Why else would he be speeding up my delivery date? But the doctor assured me there was no reason for alarm. My already soon-to-arrive son was simply ready to come into the world a bit ahead of schedule. It was something to do with test results and fluid levels. Dr. Diamond finished the non-routine, routine appointment, then handed me over to Nurse Jerry to walk me from the hospital-adjacent offices into the maternity ward. I followed her through secret hallways, through corridors I did not know existed. That day, Bryn Mawr Hospital, part of Main Line Health, felt like a maze.

"Can I call my husband? Should I re-park? I parked in the doctor's visiting area, and now...."

"Your car will be fine," Nurse Jerry promised.

She opened the heavy door to the room where I would finally meet the being that had been inside my belly for thirty-seven-and-a-half weeks.

"And you can't use your cell here."

I'd seen Nurse Jerry a lot. I'd seen my entire doctor's office staff a lot. For my third pregnancy, I'd spent week after week gazing at the zigzag lines indicating my baby's heartbeat. Each time, we failed the non-stress test. Ultrasound after ultrasound. I teased my friends that Michael and I had more photos of the baby in my tummy than of our actual children.

That day, the day the doctor decided to induce, I'd been reading *Freakonomics* to make the time pass as I waited for the results of the latest test. I was on the part about Roe v. Wade when Dr. Diamond had come into the room to inform me that my amniotic fluid was at 5.9, way too low to safely remain pregnant. I still held the book, clutched in one trembling hand, but trying to be stoic. Nurse Jerry gestured to a table. I put the book down. It wasn't until years later that I would recognize the irony of that worry-filled moment.

Roe v. Wade was the 1973 Supreme Court decision that forever changed the laws that had criminalized or restricted access to abortions. According to a CBS News August 14, 2017 online article, since prenatal screening tests were introduced in Iceland in the early 2000s, the vast majority of women—close to 100 percent—who received a positive test for Down syndrome terminated their pregnancy.

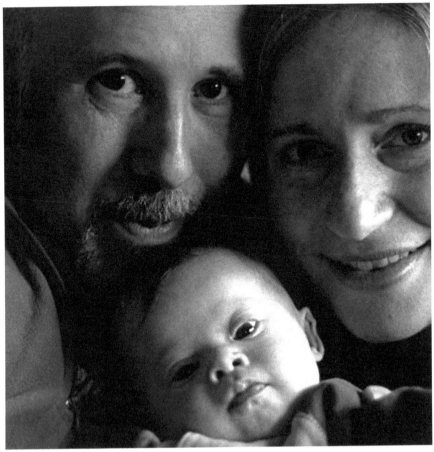

The three of us together for the first time. You can see our joy, and concern for the future here.

Looking back, while I support anyone's decision, I'm glad I didn't know about my son's genetics in advance. If I had known, I can't say for certain whether or not I'd have allowed my preconceptions and prejudices to obliterate the light and love my third boy brought, not just to me, but to all of us. Many babies with Down syndrome are aborted with no knowledge of the pure, unadulterated joy they can bring. I had no knowledge then either.

After Nurse Jerry handed me off to a labor and delivery nurse, in the hospital ward, I was given a gown and told to relax. I was already relaxed, physically. Mentally, I was doing my best not to spiral. But Dr. Diamond had assured me that they induced all the time.

A dose of Pitocin. The contractions came faster than expected. I'd had my two other sons with medication but this felt different, so I wasn't prepared for the added intensity of a labor by the medication.

Since I'd arrived at the hospital expecting a typical checkup, Michael hadn't come with me. Against Nurse Jerry's earlier admonitions, I tried calling him on the hospital phone repeatedly, but he was nowhere to be found.

No one answered at my dentist's office either.

I was supposed to have a dentist appointment after my "routine" doctor's visit. I left a message, "Sorry; I will not be at my dental exam; I am having a baby instead."

The dentist office staff later told me they had found my words hilarious. They saved my voicemail. For years, they would replay it any time they needed a laugh.

After Michael and the dentist, I phoned my friend, Trish, and cancelled my lunch plans with her. Trish was, and is, a phenomenal friend. She survived breast cancer. She inspired me with her strength, beauty, and kindness.

When Trish was going through chemotherapy, she decided to give my family her heavy, dark wood dining room table and chairs. Tom, her husband, helped her carry it all into our home. When I asked her why she was being so generous, especially at a time when she was suffering, Trish said she knew our table, a hand-me-down from my grandparents in Minnesota, got crumbs stuck in the cracks.

"Mine has no cracks for crumbs," she said. "Besides, we're getting a new set—one that isn't so heavy."

Heavy. My heart sank for what Trish was enduring, but she refused to be anything other than optimistic. Through her example, she taught me that experiences don't cause emotions. It's how we interpret what happens that determines how we feel.

I was feeling annoyed. Where was Michael? I didn't want to give birth alone. And having never had a drug-induced delivery this painful, I didn't know how long I'd be in labor.

I dialed my friend Jamie's number on the rotary hospital phone. Nurses had started coming in and out at intervals, and I didn't want them yelling at me for violating any of the hospital's phone policies.

Luckily, Jamie answered. Jamie always answered.

I had met Jamie, a friend and fellow mom, during a prenatal yoga class, taught by Gail Silver at Yoga on Main yoga studio. Gail is an extraordinary yoga teacher and author. We had both been pregnant with our oldest boys, me with Josh, she with her son Aidan. Through the years, our friendship had evolved into a rock-solid, unbreakable bond. We listened to each other's thoughts and feelings, made time to regularly connect, and supported one another through the typical ups and downs of everyday existence.

As I waited, alone, hoping Michael would pause long enough in his workday to listen to my voicemail and hurry over to the hospital, everything felt colder than it should be. I shivered. I had given birth at Bryn Mawr Hospital twice before and remembered the rooms being warmer.

Jamie appeared. "Hey, Nancy."

"Hey, Jamie. Thanks for coming." At her presence, my heart calmed. I could've sworn the room got warmer.

She reached out a reassuring hand.

I'd just started telling Jamie about the reason the doctor had decided to induce when her wind-chime ringtone went off. She checked the screen but didn't answer. I appreciated being the center of attention. That was one thing I'd long since learned about motherhood. I was almost never the most important person in the room. Few people asked about my wants, needs, and urges.

Speaking of urges, I had an overwhelming impulse to relieve myself, but the nurses had informed me earlier that I wasn't allowed out of bed. I was supposed to pee in a commode.

I couldn't go with Jamie hovering over me.

"Are you okay, Nancy?" my friend asked.

I explained my predicament.

She fetched a bedpan, then closed herself in the bathroom to quickly return her brother's call, the one she'd missed while listening to me. It took me a second to figure out why Jamie had opted for the bathroom when she could've just gone into the hall to give me the privacy I needed to pee. Then, I recalled Nurse Jerry and the others' no-cellphone policy. Jamie was smart to steer clear of the prying eyes of any hospital workers who'd have lectured her and made her end her call.

By myself in the room that had struck me as unforgivably frigid before my friend's arrival, I was able to let go and go, but, even though the relief was immediate, I was squeamish at the awkwardness of peeing while lying down. Doing things differently than usual—I didn't know then that that would become a metaphor for so many things involving my third son.

The nurse returned to the room. A cellphone-less Jamie emerged from the bathroom. My monitor must have inadvertently slipped off during my sideways commode activity, so the nurse reattached it and then applied Cervidil while Jamie averted her gaze. I flinched. Cervidil, when applied internally, can help dilate the uterus's opening. It felt like having a car part inserted in my most private area.

Just then, Michael appeared. I glared at him, a bit unfairly. He'd been at work, after all, and he was as unprepared for our third son's delivery as I was. Nevertheless, it bothered me that my husband could wander in and out of the experience, whereas I was stuck. There was no coming late or getting out early for me.

Between contractions, I watched mindless television. I've never been much of a TV person, but I needed a way to pass the time. *Three's Company* made me laugh. But, other than that, things were fairly boring. Not much seemed to be happening. I waited. Waited. Waited. The nurse brought me an Ambien. I slept. The sun came up. That was when they gave me a second dose of Pitocin. A shockwave of sensation. Contractions. Movement. I cried, although not yet from the pain, and not for a specific reason. I was overwhelmed in a general way.

When Michael asked why I was sobbing, I didn't know. Tears were simply rising from within in a giant tidal wave. Later, given what I discovered about the meaning of my third son's Hebrew name (Alexander *Gal* means ocean wave), I'd find this ironic.

At the time, though, I was too teary to contemplate ironies. And too pensive. My mind raced with all that lay ahead. All I hadn't done. I'd assumed I had more time before giving birth, and nothing felt exactly ready. Home was a jumble of undone chores.

Meanwhile, Michael couldn't stop complaining. He hadn't fed the dog or cat. His parents needed the car seats for our boys. A list of things he needed to take care of that he could have done before. Seriously? Evidently, the thought of doing for a few hours what I did every day was stressing him out. I grimaced as another contraction hit.

"Relax," he said.

I hated all three times I was in labor and my husband or the nurses told me to relax.

"I'll be back."

Really, Michael, you're leaving now?

I took a deep breath. Michael had to help his parents get our other two boys settled at home. I understood, but I wished he could stay. I love my husband and, despite my irrational, in-labor anger, I wanted him by my side.

A few moments later, he returned with a giant, sky-colored, satin-footed bear. The nurse remarked what a great guy he was. Never mind the love. The anger was back. I found myself wishing he could have the baby come out of him. A contraction. Then another. I screamed. I cried some more. Now, the pain was excruciating.

Nurse Ann walked in. "Breathe," she told me, "and relax."

There was that word again. She was trying to be helpful, but I wanted to yell at her. The pain seemed unending. Because of the Pitocin, the contractions I was experiencing were more severe than during either of the other deliveries.

The anesthesiologist arrived. I felt a sudden flash of fear. An epidural was about to be inserted into my spine. My mind rattled off a litany of possible side-effects. Another contraction. Just that quickly, I didn't care about the risks. If they had been offering crystal meth or heroin, I would have taken it.

"Stay still," the anesthesiologist soothed.

Still? How was I supposed to do that with pain coursing through me? Wave upon wave of excruciating angst that felt impossible to surf. I've never been a surfer, but I once read that the only way to ride a wave is to lean into it. I did as the anesthesiologist ordered. I didn't want to be paralyzed for life. Despite my stillness, it didn't work. They pricked me a second time while I hugged a pillow and squeezed Nurse Ann's hand. She used the dreaded R-word, "relax," again. This time, I barely cared. She was just trying to help.

Jamie was long gone by then—she'd left shortly after Michael arrived—but I harnessed my inner prenatal yogi, putting into practice the lessons I'd learned six years before when she and I had met. It worked. The second epidural was effective.

Michael reappeared. He'd been at our house for an hour.

I kicked him out. My hormones were raging, and my emotions were up, and down.

Nurse Ann checked me. The epidural continued working its magic.

I asked her to bring Michael back in. He took my hand. Squeezed. We'd been together long enough to know one another's eccentricities. To forgive and let go.

He wiped a sweaty wisp of hair from my forehead.

The end was less excruciating than the beginning. I was at ten centimeters.

Nurse Ann hurried off to get my doctor, Dr. Crate. She was kind-hearted and had a calm, easeful way about her. I appreciated her serene confidence.

"How're you doing, Nancy?" she asked.

The pain had subsided enough for me to smile. A young resident, Shannon, had accompanied the doctor into the room. She spoke to her about details and dilation. I half-expected her to reach out right then and there, and receive my third baby boy into the world, but Dr. Crate said it might take as many as eight more hours.

I was skeptical. I was also, it turned out, right. My baby boy was as eager to meet me as I was to meet him. Not an hour later, the same doctor told me to hold my knees and push.

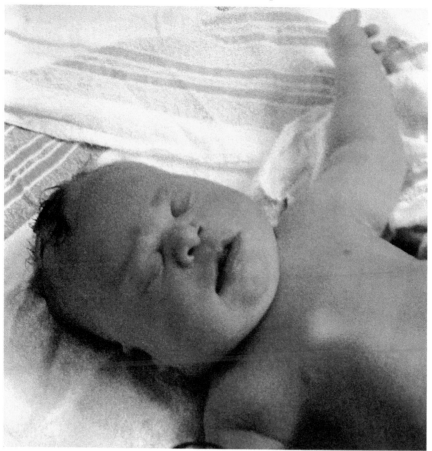

Alex's first photo. He is one minute old here. He would remain in the NICU for one month.

Alex:

What is going on? Why do Mom and Dad look so shocked, and sad? Why are they crying? Why is the doctor talking to them and holding Mom's hand? I want to snuggle Mom and Dad. Where are these people taking me? I am cold. I miss swimming inside that other place, and being with Mom. It is sterile here. I don't hear the soccer ball bouncing like at home. There are no dogs barking or cats meowing. Where am I? This bed is tiny. I miss Mom.

Finally! Mom, please don't let those nurses take me back there. The babies cry, and I miss you and Dad. Those beeps drive me batty. I am hungry. Please cuddle me, feed me. Please love me as much as I love you!

1 Shock

Despite its difficulties, this labor was the easiest of all three boys. Well, maybe not the labor. That was hard. But, with Josh and Sam, the delivery was excruciating. It took forever, and the pushing was agonizing. I almost couldn't bear it. With Alex, all that was required were a few pushes, and he was out.

His shoulders were out. He was on my belly.

Internally, I danced. I realized that, externally, something was terribly wrong. The nurses took him from me. Suddenly, a quiet deafening fell over the room... like first snow. Ten years later, as I edit this passage, it is snowing outside. I've come to understand that the tranquility that precedes what we view as a storm can also be nature's quiet acknowledgment of a new, innocent beginning. I've come to understand a lot about the wonder of the unexpected, and sometimes inconvenient. But we cannot know life's later lessons in the moment. We can only be where we are.

My heart went into freefall. It landed, with a thud, in my gut.

What was going on? I was desperate to know, and, at the same time, I didn't want to. I wanted to keep dancing. I wanted to bask in the accomplished glow of afterbirth.

Dr. Crate reached for my hand. Held it. "His ears, eyes, and neck are characteristic of Down babies."

Down what? As I tried, poorly, to process the word, it felt as if the doctor were speaking from miles away. I strained to listen through the distance. Facts. Figures. Intermittent words. Statistics. A wave of fearful questions.

I wondered about all of those weeks lying there, getting ultrasound after ultrasound. Did the doctor know ahead of time that something was wrong with my third son? If so, why hadn't he told me? I'd thought all the additional monitoring had to do with the fact that I was forty—an advanced maternal age—and, therefore, needed closer supervision.

Supervision. I would have to look after, a baby who was.... My mind roved its recesses for a way to think about my third son, but I had not yet acquired the language to explain.

Trisomy 21 is Alex's diagnosis. The medical designation refers to a chromosomal anomaly that causes a distinctive set of physical characteristics and lifelong challenges. Trisomy 21 impacts approximately 5,000 of the babies born every year. I didn't know that then. I didn't know so many things. I felt like the only one in the world with a child who would fail to live up to all the hopes and dreams I'd had for him.

How could I love an imperfect child? How did my body produce this unlovable baby? How could we live our lives in the face of this soul-crushing information? I was devastated. I didn't know how to continue living when all my dreams for my youngest were slowly withering within me.

This son would not be cute. He would be the opposite. It must be Michael's fault for using cannabis. That conviction led to our biggest argument. Ridiculous now, thinking back.

It's especially ironic considering that, years later, after Alex was diagnosed with epilepsy, I would fight to get his neurologist to agree to treat him with medical marijuana oil, instead of pharmaceutical drugs.

Sadness was like quicksand, pulling me downward. But then I had a sudden, unexpected, thought. I remembered a boy from my teaching job at Wayne Elementary School. An adorable, intelligent, and amazing young boy who had Down syndrome. The entire previous year, he'd stopped by my room to say, "Hi, Mrs. Schwartz!"

George. As far as I could tell, no obstacle had ever stopped him. I recalled him telling me about all his activities: swimming, spending time with friends, traveling to Russia, going to parties, and achieving academic success.

Even though the image of a young, smiling George calmed my heart, I was reluctant to accept that there might be something "wrong" with my own child. Michael too. We didn't capture the moment. We didn't take a photo, like we did after our other two boys' births.

Instead, I studied the purple baby.

It would be three years until Alex's baby announcement went out. Not because we needed three years to be happy about his presence, but because we were busy with the details of having a child with challenges, therapies, medicine, school meetings, and life. Plus, the demands of raising two other boys, and trying to stay married while working full-time, and trying to look good by going to the gym. I didn't know then how life would be enriched and accelerated. I understood only that I'd given birth to an abnormal baby.

There was no time to attempt to nurse Alex. No snuggling my newly-arrived third son. Instead, the nurses cleaned me up. Checked the baby. Carted him off. Michael and I were left alone with our shock. Quiet. No words. No celebration.

After checking our baby, Dr. Kapper, a neonatologist, confirmed Dr. Crate's observations about Alex's neck, eyes, and ears. I recalled how, after their births, the doctor handed my other two sons to me. Michael and I were left alone to savor. This felt like the wrong ending to a story. As if what I'd thought would be a happily-ever-after fairytale had turned out, instead, to be a tragedy.

I was taken from the delivery room to my own private recovery room. I cried. Michael cried. The last time I'd seen him cry had been on June 6, 1995, the day his brother, Barry, died.

Using the rotary phone provided by the hospital, I called every friend I could think of. I told everyone who answered that we'd had a baby boy; then I quickly staunched the flow of their excitement with the announcement that my third son, whose perfect arrival I had taken for granted, had Down syndrome. My friends were far more circumspect than I. By and large, they validated my confusion and disappointment while reminding me not to project too far into the future.

"You don't know what this means yet," they told me. "Or how raising him will be. Try not to get down about it. Try to keep your spirits up."

My son, they said, might have come in unconventional wrapping paper, but he was nevertheless a gift.

Finally, a nurse came into my new room with my infant son swaddled in her arms. I was united with the baby. No, not *the* baby. *Our* baby. Alex.

Alex wasn't with me for long. While I stayed in my room, he was taken back to the Neonatal Intensive Care Unit (NICU).

The NICU was a foreign country. Beeps. Wires. Nurses with serious expressions. Doctors checking computers. Miniature beds with babies small enough to hold in the palm of my hand. Heart monitors and ringing alarms. Beeping oxygen, and pulse ox monitors. The interminable buzzing of machines. Medicines, screens, strange sounds.... I will never forget those sounds. It was like New York City at rush hour.

And, then, there he was, with a tube in his nose. My little boy. Looking back now, I can't help but wonder why it took me so long to see what now seems self-evident.

It wasn't until visiting Alex in the NICU that the surge of love I'd felt immediately upon seeing Josh and Sam welled up within me. But, even then, my emotions remained tainted. It took my other boys to teach me how to love Alex without judgment.

When he saw his younger brother for the first time, Sam was far from repulsed.

"He is the cutest baby in the world," he told his father and me. And my heart cracked open. Sam was right, I realized. And even though I wasn't ready to completely adopt a different way of looking at our situation, his words buoyed my heart and lifted my spirits. His words opened my eyes to the possibility that there might be an upside to Alex's Down syndrome.

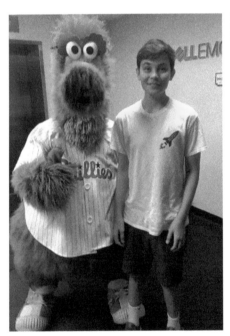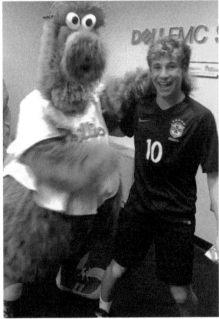

Josh Schwartz, Sam Schwartz, and the Phillie Phanatic at the Philadelphia Phillies Stadium

A nasal cannula helped deliver oxygen to Alex's lungs. Why couldn't he just take a deep breath and be okay? I had an urge to pick him up and take him home. We could all continue our lives. Why did all these medical people have to be involved? I craved everything to be as it was. Well, not as it was, but as I was beginning to let myself hope it could be.

In addition to Sam's eye-opening words, knowing my youngest son's life was in danger had catapulted me out of wishing he were different into simply wanting him to be safe.

I hadn't expected to leave Bryn Mawr Hospital without my baby, and the inner ache was almost intolerable. I had a hard time parting with Alex, even for an hour. Who am I kidding? Even for a minute. I would briefly go home to attend to the other boys, shower, change, throw in a load of laundry. Funny how I found myself envying a setting on a dryer. Normal. If only....

Every time I left, I longed to carry Alex out of the hospital to our bustling home. Every time I got home, I'd miss him so much I couldn't stay. I'd rush back, desperate for even a few seconds with my youngest son.

I craved each and every typical mother-infant interaction. Trying to ignore the alien wires protruding out of my strong, struggling son, I would hold him to my breast while praying that he might be as hungry for what I had to offer as I was to give.

In the NICU, a lactation expert, Terry, explained to Michael and me, beeps interrupting her every word, "You have to feed him sideways to help him organize for the milk you pumped." Terry explained that due to his genetics, Alex would have a harder time settling to eat. To this day, her words remain true. At mealtimes, my youngest often gets distracted. He'll need to pause between bites in order to breathe or to have a sip of water before continuing to eat.

Michael was better at holding and feeding Alex than I was. The ways I had to modify for Alex didn't feel intuitive to me, and my upper arm strength was non-existent. Oh, how my arms have changed. We sometimes joke that I have acquired the same brute force that allows people to lift cars off victims. Hero strength. Mother strength. I am more powerful than I've ever been. All because the son I once thought of as a liability has taught me the asset of having to do things differently. He has taught me to harness my physical and emotional resilience.

It's ten years later, and I'm pretty sure I could qualify for a competitive weightlifting competition just from the daily training that mothering Alex provides. I intend to lift him as long as I can.

My third grade ELL (English Language Learning) student, Young, is a cousin of the renowned violinist, Sara Chang. Young proudly regales the class with stories of his talented cousin. Recently, he told us that even while suffering from terrible neck pain, Sara kept playing her violin for six straight hours.

"How'd she do that?" a fellow student wanted to know.

"She loves it that much," Young replied.

I love Alex that much. I have trained my body to carry him, yet it feels as if he is the one carrying me.

When she met Alex, my niece, Rivka, prophesized, "Aunt Nancy, this little boy will make you strong."

He has. He has helped all of us to develop a level of resilience we never knew we had.

Before Alex was born, Michael and I would have never thought to expose Josh or Sam to life's precariousness. We shielded them because we were blind to the incredibly uplifting potential of some of life's downsides and difficulties. Then, their brother, arrived.

We regularly brought Josh and Sam to the NICU. I bit back tears when they wondered why Alex couldn't come home to the mint-green bassinet with puffy stars hanging on it that I'd lovingly placed beside my and Michael's bed.

"He lives in the hospital," I explained. "But not for long."

They held their baby brother and posed for photos (see next page).

Josh and Sam showed Alex the bear I'd brought in anticipation of his arrival. I took in the stuffed, furry face and was transported back to a time, months earlier, when, belly swollen, I'd strode into a shop in downtown Princeton and bought the softest, most comforting thing I could find. As I stood, shivering, in the impersonal NICU, there was no comfort to be found in inanimate objects—only in the slow rise and fall of my youngest's chest, and in the unwavering trust of his two older brothers. Josh and Sam weren't scared. They were impatient. They knew without a doubt that Alex would be coming home. They merely didn't want to wait.

"We didn't bring the letters," Sam informed me.

It took a minute for my scared, and scattered, brain to figure out what he was referring to. At the same Princeton shop where I'd

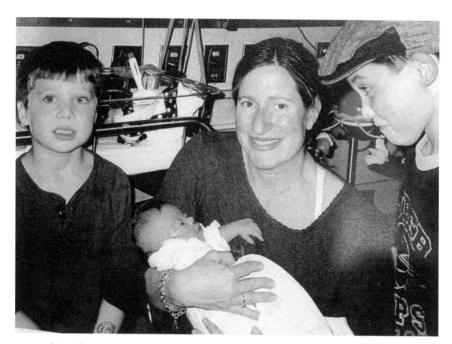

One of the first photos of me with my three boys the month Alex spent in the NICU (Neonatal Intensive Care Unit).

gotten the bear, I'd bought four colorful, animal-shaped wooden letters. The letters, which spelled out A L E X, were already hanging on Alex's designated bedroom door, waiting, under the letters S A M. When Alex did finally join us, in his new and receptive home, he and Sam would share a room. Well, after Michael and I let go of the need to keep Alex in with us. It was as if I wanted to make up for all the forced separation. But I didn't know then, as I stood in the NICU, that I would hover over Alex like a helicopter. Didn't know yet that mothering him would require more from me than I'd have believed possible.

I said a silent prayer of thanks that Sam wanted to share. My son the citizen, never territorial, always eager to include.

For a while, the NICU became our family's second home. I spent more hours camped out by Alex's side than anywhere else. I learned the names of all the nurses, for all the shifts, and exchanged worried glances with other nervous parents.

Up until Alex's arrival, I had been terrified of all things medical. At age ten, I had to have my thyroid taken out. As my parents drove around and around the circular parking garage, I hoped desperately that they wouldn't find a spot. If they couldn't park the car, I thought the doctors couldn't operate. I didn't understand anesthesia, and I was terrified of having my neck sliced open.

It wasn't long before I became accustomed to the hospital. I spoke Vietnamese to the man who helped clean. I watched the nurses perform their tiny daily miracles. I snuggled Alex. Held his hand. I remember thinking that if I held his hand, he would know I loved him. I sang songs, and read books. I read him *Guess How Much I Love You* by Sam McBratney so many times I memorized each and every word. I showed Anita Jeram's beautiful illustrations to Alex.

I knew from the literature I'd read and from what the doctors told me that infants can't see color, but I didn't care. I wanted to forge a connection. Plus, I was convinced my third son could understand my words.

With each passing day, this conviction has grown stronger. Alex hears me. Sometimes, when I tell people this, they smile indulgently, their disbelief clear, but I know my son has always been a sponge, absorbing and retaining. Even if he can't express.

My friend, Brucie, who also has a son with challenges, told me that she, too, knew her son took things in. She affirmed truths I held within myself and gave me insights I hadn't had before.

The hospital paperwork was overwhelming. It seemed as if even the forms had forms. When I wasn't helicoptering over Alex, chatting with other anxious parents, or quizzing the nurses about my son's medical status, I was signing on the dotted line and providing yet another treatment consent.

Thankfully, Alex had been assigned a phenomenal social worker. I knew right away that we'd lucked out with Liz Bland. A dynamic mix of practical and empathetic, she was able to help me navigate my feelings while offering valuable facts. There was so much I didn't know. So many questions. Yet, Liz never seemed to tire of my inquiries. She met my persistence with patience. She was someone I could count on. I still count on her. She's no longer Alex's social worker, but we stay in touch through social media, and she's made it clear that she's only ever a phone call away.

"You can't make him breathe," she told me in the early days following Alex's birth, the days where I didn't know if he would live or die.

Intellectually, her reminder struck me as self-evident. Alex's breathing capacity was out of my control. So much was out of my control. I needed to take care of myself and trust the doctors with my precious son. But within me surged a tidal wave of terror.

After we gave Alex his name (Alexander Gunnar Gal Schwartz), several friends commented about the symbolic meaning: *Gal* is Hebrew for ocean wave. Alex was exactly that. Magnificent and full of life, surging with surprises, and lapping love upon my shores. Still, worry eroded my insides.

One gray, rainy day, I found myself crying on Liz's shoulder. I wanted Alex at home in the room with the letters on the door. Instead of talking to me about my son's prognosis, she told me to take time each day for myself.

"Get your nails or your toes done," she advised. "Sit with a latte. Take care of yourself."

Wise words. To this day, I follow her advice.

The giant picture windows at the hospital let the light in. The NICU was in the basement where it was darker. When it was cloudy, and raining, I felt like my heart might stop if I remained there too long. It was not seasonal affective disorder. It was a need to see light. I searched for it not just outside but everywhere, and the absence of it physically hurt. Funny because Alex exudes light. Perhaps I should've looked to him more, but I was still laboring under the misconception that he needed us more than we needed him. I would eventually realize just how distorted this thinking was, but I hadn't yet come to see Alex's challenges as the source of so many blessings. I was too focused on my own insecurity as well as on inconveniences and logistics.

Everyone who visited the NICU had to scrub their hands clean to the elbow. Every time I went to see Alex, which was every day, I felt completely out of sorts. Sometimes, it was as bad as being on a boat in the middle of a storm. I'd feel nauseous.

This isn't where I wanted to be, I'd think. Especially not with my baby. Our baby.

But I also didn't want to be anywhere other than by Alex's side. I cried a lot in those days. I wished Michael would cry too, but he remained stoic. We were each grieving in our own ways—shared feelings with different modes of expression. I found myself wishing, sometimes, for a translator to help us better understand each other. Little did I know...Alex would prove to be just that.

Magically, friends appeared at the NICU helping to erase the fear, and pain of the unknown. People I thought long gone from my life....

Andrea, a friend I met during a shared geology class in college, brought Hope's Cookies, a delicious brand of gourmet cookies that offered sweet comfort. Beth and Trish brought scented body oils from Whole Foods. I inhaled their aromas and felt a reawakening of sensory sensations. I hadn't realized how closed off I'd been from my body, how focused on the sensations I imagined were occurring within my son. I thought about yoga. The union of breath and movement. I knew I needed to do a better job of leading by example. Leading with love.

Fear is a closed door. Love is the key that opens it.

Throughout the parade of my friends, my husband was silent. His cellphone remained in his pocket, closed. Like his heart. No calls to friends. No reaching out for information or support. No laughter. No joy. Just fear. Occasional tears of uncertainty. But he'd mostly shed these when he couldn't help himself or when he was alone. I'd walk into a room and catch him wiping his eyes, but he refused to open up. Even to me.

I was beside myself. Clearly, Michael was hurting. Why wouldn't he do something to help himself? And, if he refused to do that, why couldn't he snap out of it?

I realize now that we all handle loss, change, and grief differently. One way isn't any more right than another. We bring our own unique paintbrushes to our canvas of life.

Ironically, it was Alex who taught me that.

Michael did call several of his friends after giving the reality of Alex's birth time to set in. I couldn't make him ready to share, nor should I have tried. It's strange how it took having a son for whom everything requires a different perspective for me to be willing to accept the differences in those without designated, culturally recognized challenges. I say that because we all have challenges. It's part of what makes life a rich, and wonderful tapestry.

The truth is, I should've been worrying less about how my husband chose to navigate the logistics of our perceived loss. I should've worried less, period.

In the coming days, weeks, months, and years, Alex would help me dig deeply and discover courage and acceptance. He would help me find glimpses of wisdom.

As for Michael, his friends supported him too. When he did reach out, a week or so after our youngest's arrival into the world, he told them about Alex, and they visited the NICU.

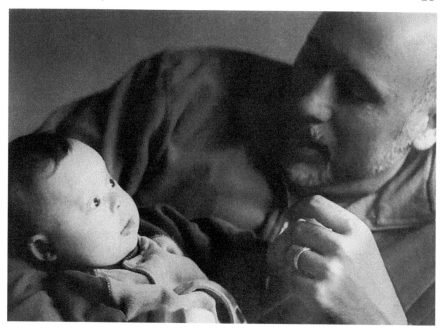

You can see the love Michael and Alex share here in this early photo.

To give you a sense of how incomprehensible Michael's behavior was to me, I should explain I am a divulger of information. I share feelings and facts. I've always craved closeness with others and, even before Alex's arrival, I had amassed a network of connections with whom I spoke regularly. As soon as the doctor broke the then-heart-wrenching, now life-affirming, news that my third son would be a challenged child, I began reaching out.

My broken voice vacillated between tears of happiness, and tears of terror as I spoke into the hospital's landline receiver. "We had a baby boy," I told friend after friend. I have to tell the news quickly, like ripping off a Band-Aid. "He was born with Down syndrome." I needed to say it upfront, to remind myself of what was true, and to prevent the pain of a slow, excruciating disclosure.

I didn't want people going too far down the path of congratulations until they understood that this situation was tinged with ambivalence. Again, I was wanting to control others' reactions. I didn't realize it at the time, but I was projecting my own secretly harbored insecurities, judgments, and prejudices onto others. I had developed many false beliefs about what it meant to be born with a disability, and about what the parents of such children might have to "endure." It strikes me as silly now that I would think my situation was so dire when, in fact, our lives were enriched by Alex almost from the outset. In retrospect, maybe Michael was onto something in waiting to process his feelings before opening up about them. A week after Alex's arrival, my feelings were far more accepting than in those early hours and days after his birth, and they would continue to morph—from shock to horror to tolerance to acceptance to curiosity to enlightenment to the unmitigated joy that I have been blessed with three tremendous sons, the last of whom has helped my soul grow in ways I never knew it needed to.

Still, I'm grateful I shared so much, and with so many, following Alex's birth. I needed others to hold a mirror up to the situation, to reflect, to refract my limited vision, and to help me see a fuller version of the picture.

My friend, Elizabeth Castiglione, has an openness and a purity of heart I desperately needed when I was still reeling from the after-shock of the "His ears, eyes, and neck are characteristic of Down babies" earthquake. She told me I looked like an earth mother, and that Alex, too, was beautiful. And she gently reminded me of her birthday, which, it so happened, was the week of Alex's birthday too.

I couldn't help but smile at that connection. Elizabeth always speaks her truth, and her artistic gift colors the world with beauty. I was inspired to know Alex shared a birthday with her.

Deidre, another friend, later told me she thought it took courage for me to call people. But it was people like her who gave me the courage to go on, to lean into my faith and stay open enough that I was quickly able to love Alex and rejoice in what I'd previously thought was an intolerable situation. Deidre and her husband Bob made sure I was able to attend a talk by my favorite rabbi, Rabbi Wolpe. They were generous enough to pay for my ticket.

Rabbi Wolpe was speaking at my old Hebrew High School, Akiba, about his book, *Why Faith Matters*, the night before Alex came home.

With Josh and Sam, people cared about the new additions to our family but aside from congratulatory cards, a smattering of calls, and a guest or two, Michael and I were largely left alone to handle our parenting obligations. We certainly never had a seemingly endless stream of visitors when we had Josh and Sam. My International Parent Group, my book group, my work friends, family members,

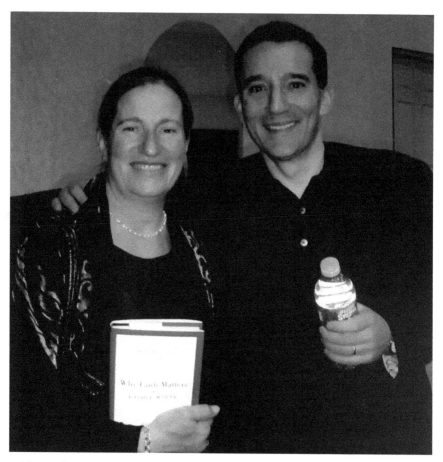

Rabbi Wolpe and me the night before Alex came home from being in the NICU for a month. The event was for his book release, *Why Faith Matters*. Deidre and Bob made this happen. I will always be thankful to them for inspiring my faith.

and other friends all arrived in droves, each bringing a gift of love. From the time Alex was in the NICU through the first several months after we brought Alex home, loved ones showed up and supported us. They fastidiously scrubbed their hands and arms so they could hold Alex. And during the month he was in the NICU, many of them met me for coffee. Their hope was what I needed. I clutched it to me like a life raft. I clutched whatever I could grab hold of that would tether me to my newfound reality and help me feel a sense of purpose amid my inner powerlessness.

The month Alex spent in the hospital felt endless. It felt like all the other babies got to leave, but not ours. As much as I admired and respected the NICU nurses and staff, I just wanted to bring my baby home. Nothing about his birth felt "normal," but I labored under the belief that having Alex at home, out of the hospital, would be the answer to the heaviness in my heart.

It's bittersweet to think about that time now that Alex is ten and Michael and I have been providing him with constant care while trying desperately to get at-home assistance.

Even in the midst of my conviction that I, a non-medical professional with no knowledge about, or meaningful experience of Down syndrome was the best equipped to offer care for my son, the NICU nurses continued to amaze me with their skills. They dressed Alex in adorable outfits, taking time to cover his head in matching hand-made warm fuzzy hats that coordinated perfectly with the rest of his clothes.

I'd watch the nurses change the incubator bedding while holding its former tiny occupant. If alarms sounded from heart or oxygen machines, they kept their composure, never letting on the danger that each baby faced. They emailed each day to provide updates on how each baby was. I rarely needed email updates since I was almost always there. They made sure doctors were notified and kept track of where each physician needed to be for any emergent situation. The nurses monitored feeding tubes, read reports, noted changes, communicated with parents and staff, and acted as angels on earth.

Donna, one of the nurses, told me that even though Alex couldn't articulate what he wanted, she could tell from his behavior that he liked to be warm. I thought of her as a "baby whisperer" and was glad to have my son being looked after by someone so attentive and perceptive.

Later, after realizing the full joy and beauty Alex brought, and continues to bring, to our lives, I wished I had been more celebratory at my third son's arrival. Reading through his thick medical report as I prepared to write this memoir, I was reminded that it wasn't merely shock, and disappointment that made it hard to rejoice. Alex's early life was precarious.

In that medical report, I saw something I never knew. He had to be resuscitated. No one told me. And, yet, instead of being angry they hadn't kept me apprised, I'm grateful. I'm glad I didn't know at the moment it happened. I lived in daily fear that Alex might die, and any confirmation of his fragility would have devastated me. I needed to borrow Josh and Sam's unwavering belief. They *knew* their brother was okay. Michael didn't know, but he suspected. Or, at least, he tried to put on a brave front.

I struggled to be brave.

I wished I could absorb all of Alex's difficulties into myself. Wished my love could be like oxygen, suffusing his tiny lungs with the air of adoration. Sometimes, I'd be watching him unable to breathe and find I had forgotten to inhale. I reminded myself of all the friends, relatives, nurses, doctors, and social workers who told me, emphatically, that the best way to mother Alex—and Josh and Sam—was to nurture myself first.

I tried. Luckily, when I faltered, my circle of support was constantly there. Friends visited regularly. Our next-door neighbors, Carol, Kevin, and Joe, brought us delicious Italian food. Whether we asked or not, people showed up to help. I desperately needed these outside reminders of life outside of a sterile, antiseptic environment.

Time in the hospital moved at a strange pace. On sunny days, the NICU was an easier place for me to be than on more inclement days. The weather seemed to deeply affect my mood. I still don't know why. In retrospect, I think it had something to do with needing an infusion of hope from the external elements because my inner ability to find joy felt uncertain.

In the hospital, a nurse gave me a book on Down syndrome. I could not open it. I did not want to see the pictures. I could not bring myself to look at the faces. It all struck me as a reminder of how my life had been ruined.

But was it?

The visit that most imprinted itself on my soul, which I can recall so vividly that even as I write these words, ten years later, I can still conjure up the experience, was a visit from Grace. Grace is a perfect name for my elegant friend. A stunning woman full of positive vibes, and good karma, she appeared at the hospital on the second day of Alex's life, clad in jeans and dock sliders with perfectly coiffed hair. I was in a hospital gown, blood still oozing from the birth.

Nevertheless, Michael and I led her downstairs to the NICU. She took one look at Alex and said how cute he was. She wouldn't even entertain the idea that he was anything other than exactly as he should be.

"He has ten tiny toes and fingers," she pointed out. Then, she reminded me about George, the boy who had stopped by my classroom each day the previous year. Jenny, a book group friend, had told Grace how much George had meant to me, and Grace had not only retained the information but had stored specific memories of my memories, as told to her by someone else. Her kind and gentle reminders helped reorient me out of pity into a sense of possibility. I found myself grateful for Jenny, too. She knew the power in speaking to others as we journey along our path. These women held me up to the light at a time where darkness threatened to take my days.

Grace would become one of my pillars of strength and a true model for how I want to live my life. I should say also that Grace is George's mom. She knew firsthand what it was to have a challenged child. I always thought Grace was a pillar of strength in spite of George, but she explained that he has been a source of inspiration. She wrote a book about mothering George, and although I didn't decide to write this book until I had more experience with Alex, as I reflect back on Grace's reflections, I see her as an enduring source of inspiration.

The days in the NICU were long, so I was thankful for Grace's visit—and everyone's visits—but Grace's in particular because she had something none of the others did: direct experience. Not only did she break up the monotony, but she offered a different perspective, one I desperately needed at the time. A perspective based on her personal experience, strength, and hope.

The day following her NICU visit, Grace called to check in on me. Through tears that came so fast and hard I nearly choked on them, I explained that my life felt upside down. Grace, calm as a lake in my mom's native Minnesota, said, "Let me tell you what my dad told me. People will respond to him the way you respond to him. He is an addition. That's it. He's not anything other than an addition."

She was speaking about what her father had said after George's birth.

I nodded.

She continued. "He is not taking anything away from Josh or Sam. Say the Serenity Prayer: G-d, grant me the serenity to accept the things I cannot change, the courage to change the things I can, and the wisdom to know the difference."

Her spiritual surety was a balm for my heart. I took her words into me as a salve. I wrote them down. My wounded soul began to heal.

Years later, Grace's sentiments still carry the power to turn things from upside down to right side up. I kept those words on that yellow NICU notepaper. I carry those words still, ten years later, in my heart. And I've said the Serenity Prayer so many times that, in times of strife, it rises unbidden to the surface, washing over me in a gentle wave. A gentle wave...Alexander Gal. Without my youngest son in my life, I would never have learned about the serenity that comes with surrender.

As time passed, Grace continued to help me with her wisdom.

"Be happy, totally happy," she advised. "Celebrate every day; make holidays special; decorate.... Distract yourself and be up. Get Alex a cute haircut. Always dress him well."

She lent me the books *Simple Abundance* by Sara Ban Breathnach, and *Chicken Soup for the Mother's Soul* by Jack Canfield, Mark Victor Hansen, Jennifer Read Hawthorne, and Marci Shimoff. Those books shaped my ability to move through motherhood and life differently. In *Simple Abundance*, I read how keeping a comfort drawer can change your life. I created one. I filled a drawer with bubble bath that smelled like strawberry, fancy soaps that were tied with beautiful satin ribbons, and expensive chocolates to savor. This drawer was always available. That way, whenever a day came that I needed some extreme self-care, there it was. In *Chicken Soup for the Mother's Soul,* the authors highlighted stories of hope conquering fear. I needed hope. I lived on hope. And, in those early days, I had trouble cultivating hope from within. External sources were necessary.

My friend, Sonya, visited me with flowers. The International Parent Group I had helped start at Wayne Elementary School came. It was humbling to see a collection of strong women showing their support and allegiance. I'd always admired the parent group members who had the resolve and resilience to leave their countries of origin to learn new customs and a new language to create lives, build families, and establish obligations. Yet, they made time to be a friend to me. For three straight months after Alex's arrival, the school where I worked, my book group, and the International Parent Group brought dinners to our home on a rotating basis. The overwhelming outpouring of tangible love fed my heart. Without it, I'm not sure how we would've functioned. But Alex opened the doors of friendship for us all in ways we never thought possible. Even as an infant, he tore down walls between people. He does it now too—so often, in fact, that I have ceased to be surprised.

Lessons Alex Taught Me:

- When you think your life as you know it is over, know that you can choose to embrace your current situation as the beginning of something wonderful.

- People (strangers, new friends, doctors, therapists, and teachers) will respond to your child the way you respond to your child.

- If you are struggling to respond to your child the way you want, it helps to lean on those you trust for invaluable insights.

- Say the Serenity Prayer every day: G-D, grant me the serenity to accept the things I cannot change, the courage to change the things I can, and the wisdom to know the difference.

- Differences can be beautiful.

- Love has no limits.

- Love creates strength.

Alex:

Where are my parents? They come every day. I hope they are coming. I miss them. I miss my brothers too. I wish Mom and Dad would stop being sad. I am happy to be here in the world. I think they are upset because of me. It does not make sense. I wish these people would take these wires off of me. I am sick of this tube in my nose with the hurricane sound of oxygen. Why is it so noisy here? The beeps are giving me a headache.

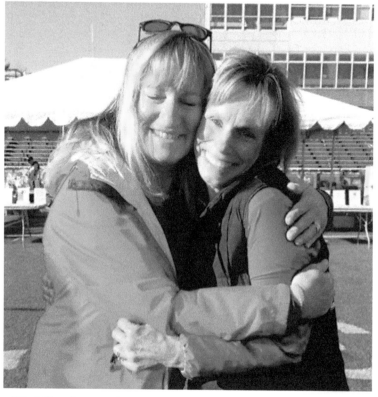

Grace Wadell and me at the Children's Hospital of Philadelphia (CHOP) Buddy Walk. She was one of the founders of this walk which made it possible to create a clinic for children with Down syndrome called "The Trisomy 21 Program" at CHOP.

2 Oxygen

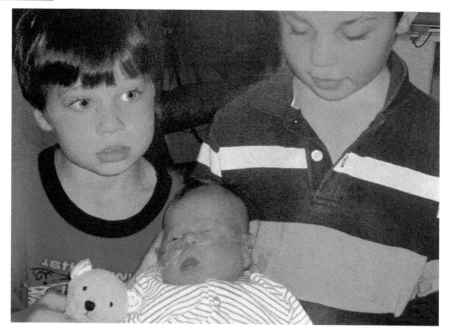

The first photo we have of our three boys together was taken in the NICU.

As you can see, Alex has a tube in his nose (aka a nasal cannula). This particular medical device had been inserted to help him grow his lungs and breathe. Alex would need oxygen for a month, and this life-giving oxygen cord both sustained his existence and tethered him to the NICU. Its necessity kept us from bringing our precious baby home.

Thinking back, I find it ironic that I view Alex himself as a source of my own spiritual oxygenation. I continue to want to breathe air in this world because of Alex. I love all my boys, of course. I cannot imagine my life without Alex, Josh, or Sam. They bring happiness to each day. Yet, my third son is dependent on me in ways the other two simply aren't. There is a way in which Alex needs me, and I need him, that has created a symbiotic relationship between us.

I am Alex's interpreter, his advocate, the decipherer of his symptoms, the tracker of his moods. And he is the architect of my soul. I breathe him in. He breathes me in. We exist because of the love we give one another.

I'm not the only one who feels this way. Even Seamus, our black-and-white Border Collie, is drawn to Alex in ways he simply isn't to the rest of us. Seamus is so sweet and soulful that it's impossible to see him as a "pet." He is a member of our family, a rare and wonderful breed of compassion and connection. If any one of us gets hurt, Seamus senses it and is quickly at our side, offering a much-needed nuzzle.

Never mind that we took Seamus to special dog obedience training for "What a good dog" lessons and the only thing he retained was how to react to the word "off," he has trained himself to be Alex's helper dog.

But all that wouldn't come until later. Until my beautiful boy was out of the immediate terror of his early infancy. In the meantime, I was Alex's helper, his impotent ally, looking on in terror as my baby struggled to breathe.

The cannula saddened me.

Alex was in the NICU a full month before they finally released him to our care. The best, and worst, part about the time he spent there was that the rest of our family had to function in the outside world. Michael, Josh, Sam, and I lived our lives. We attended a birthday party at the Morris Arboretum for Erica, the daughter of our family friends, the Waldmans. They had fairies to admire, and tree houses to climb. Our boys drank in the normalcy. I watched them and realized, not for the first time, and certainly not for the last, that I had three boys. Out of necessity, I'd been focusing on my youngest, but my eldest and middle sons needed me too. And I needed them. I'd gotten so consumed with nasal cannulas, and monitors, and beeps, and vital statistics that I'd forgotten the rest of my roles and responsibilities. Not to mention the daily joys that had been part of life before Alex and would continue to be part of life after he arrived.

The art opening for my student's mom, Josette Simon-Gestin, from Brittany, France, was a much-needed diversion. I was able to appreciate the evening and become engrossed in the exhibition. It quieted the nagging inner panic that had been with me since the Trisomy 21 diagnosis.

Life moved on, but part of my heart slept at the hospital.

Alex's situation was out of my control. I was forced to ask myself what was in my control. The answer was my actions and attitudes. The answer is always my actions and attitudes. Throughout the days and weeks I waited for my baby to come home, I found myself thinking often of a greeting card I had purchased in Maine when Michael and I were dating. The card read:

> The longer I live, the more I realize the impact of attitude on life. Attitude, to me, is more important than facts. It is more important than the past, than education, than money, than circumstances, than failures, than successes, than what other people think or say or do. The remarkable thing is we have a choice every day regarding the attitude we will embrace for that day. We cannot change our past. We cannot change the fact that people will act in a certain way. We cannot change the inevitable. The only thing we can do is play on the one string we have, and that is our attitude. I am convinced that life is 10% what happens to me, and 90% how I react to it. And so it is with you. We are in charge of our attitudes.
>
> — Charles R. Swindoll

When we nurture ourselves, we have more to give those we love. This is particularly important when caring for a child with challenges. In those early days, I had to force myself to care for myself. I was so consumed by mothering that I struggled to see myself as a separate entity with needs and desires of her own.

It's gotten easier.

After preschool, at KinderCare in Radnor, Pennsylvania, across the street from the school where I teach, I would pick up Alex. And, truth be told, if I got a break during the day, I'd sometimes sneak across the street to steal a hug from my smiling son.

Sometimes, my colleague, Teresa, accompanied me to say hi to him and receive her own hug. Even though we had reserved a spot at the preschool for Alex before he was born, I had phoned, panicked, and left a message for the director, Annette, telling her that Alex had Down syndrome and wouldn't be able to attend. She phoned back to say that, of course, he could come.

He was "more than welcome."

My son. Welcome. Her words broke my heart, and stitched it back together all at once.

After Alex attended their school, Terry, the head of the Kinder-Care, would have a nephew whose child was born with Down syndrome. Yet again, my experiences with Alex gave value to the world. I had the rare and wonderful experience of being able to talk to her nephew about the blessing of having a child like Alex.

Following his preschool days, my youngest attended Saint David's Nursery School (SDNS) where the kind director, Joanne, loved him like we did. Since Alex attended SDNS, we have encouraged other parents with children who have a Down syndrome diagnosis to send their children there.

Alex attends public school now. He loves learning and being with his friends and teachers at school.

A video posted to Instagram from his regular education teacher showed Alex and his classmates dancing to a song on the program *Go Noodle.* I could see Alex smile and try to dance from his wheelchair, which he has needed since he was born. This made my heart soar. Alex knows so much. He learns from his peers. His peers learn from him. One mom told me her daughter Mairead talks about Alex regularly. I know, if he could speak, my son would tell us about his friends, especially Mairead who showed up to his birthday party with three huge stuffed animals—an owl, a puppy, and a groundhog.

At a work meeting the other day, at the elementary school where I work, I overheard people talking disparagingly about children with challenges. One person, whom I did not know and who did not know me or my story, said something about how she "tolerates these kids."

Sometimes, when I am feeling introspective, I think back to how I felt when the hospital staff gave me a book on children with Down syndrome. I felt unable to open it because of my own ignorance and prejudice. Now, when I see pictures of children with Trisomy 21, they seem as gorgeous and rare as shooting stars. I do not see their medical diagnoses. I see their shining essences, and I hope and pray that others can see the same when they look at my son. But I know that a closed mind is a locked door, impossible to open without a key.

Alex has been my key. He has also been a key for many others who have had the chance to experience his unique spirit directly. And yet, strangers sometimes assume challenged children are burdens, as opposed to blessings.

It made me sad that many people are blind to the potential that exists in all children. Each child is a gift.

When Alex was three years old, my husband called to say, "Alex pointed to his water!" I felt an upsurge of love and pride then that I can still summon if I just close my eyes.

This was the first time Alex had been able to tell one of us he wanted water—to express a need in real-time so we didn't have to guess. My greatest hope for all my boys is that they are able to pursue their passions in life—to know what they want and move toward it. Alex may not have the capacity to verbalize yet, but the day he pointed to his water, he was showing us he had a voice, and I was moved to happy tears.

Alex continues to be full of miracles. Endless potential. Love, kindness, sweetness, goodness, and light.

Now that Alex is older, Michael and I sometimes send him to sleep over at his friend Jeffrey's home so we can have some time to focus on ourselves and maintain our relationship. I never thought Alex would be invited to other children's houses, let alone gain life-long friends. As a neurologically challenged child, I thought the only people who could love him would be us—his family. That has proven to be far from true. Although Jeffrey and Alex's friendship is beyond special, Jeffrey is not Alex's only friend. Far from it. It continues to amaze me that my third son can make friends without words. He connects to people through their hearts. He has his own communication system.

After their first sleepover, Jeffrey asked to do it again. I know that if Alex could use his voice, he would have requested the same.

When we picked him up to bring him home, he even tried to say goodbye. Since that first time beneath another family's roof, Alex has been more expressive. Even if he does not yet have conventional language skills, he has found ways to articulate his needs.

"How was it?" I asked as I collected my youngest.

Jeffrey's mom, Shannon O'Donnell Grimes, laughingly explained that, although they had a great time, Alex was not a huge fan of church.

Jeffrey's family attends Presentation Blessed Virgin Mary, a Catholic church in Wynnewood, Pennsylvania. They brought Alex along to expose him to new things because I had encouraged them to incorporate Alex into their regular routines and rituals. Once I began to experience Alex as a person, instead of a diagnosis, I became convinced that giving him a sense of belonging was essential. But more on that later.

At church, Alex signed to Shannon that he'd rather be eating dinner instead of sitting in a pew—like so many other churchgoing children, I imagine.

I smiled when Shannon told me about my son's articulated boredom. I continue to be happy each time Alex expresses his feelings and interests—or, in this case, disinterest. I want him to have a voice and to use it. And it thrills me every time my youngest is exposed to different things. Like religion. I want his world to be ever-expanding.

Michael and I and our boys are Jewish. We attend synagogue at Beth Hillel-Beth El, in Wynnewood, Pennsylvania. Alex comes with us, so he has grown used to that experience.

What Shannon told me made me hopeful for the future. I thought it was funny that Alex responded as a lot of children would: Feed me. I don't want to sit through this service.

Lessons Alex Taught Me:

- It is possible to make lifelong friends by connecting with them through the heart.
- The future is full of hope.
- The future is bright.
- Friends keep us happy, positive, and peaceful.
- Learning about others, their lives, and rituals is important.
- Taking care of one's own needs is essential.
- Just because a person cannot speak does not mean they cannot understand or communicate.
- Tolerance is not enough; we must embrace differences and accept everyone, especially children, as they are.

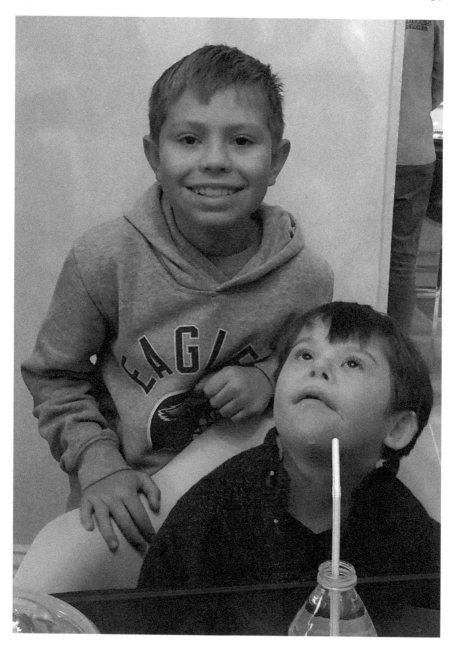

Alex and Jeffrey. Jeffrey is Alex's best friend. He was the first friend to invite Alex to his firetruck birthday party at the fire station. I never thought Alex would be invited to a birthday party when he was born. The two have been friends for over ten years.

Alex:

I am happy to be home with my family. I love them all more than I can ever say. That hospital was nice, but it is not my place. This is wonderful to be together. I love seeing my name A L E X on my door with my brother's name, S A M. Home is the best.

3

Light

We sent Alex's birth announcement three years after he was born. I was inspired to send them because of Francis Dunnery, a fabulous writer, musician, and astrologer. I went to see him for two astrology readings, and soon after that, I began listening to his inspirational music.

"You're the most beautiful thing that I ever saw in my life," are the lyrics to Francis' song, "Sunshine."

As I listened to the song, and allowed Francis' words to flow through me, I thought of Alex, Josh, and Sam—the most beautiful things I ever saw. Beauty, I have learned, does not equate to perfection.

For a long time after Alex was born, I found myself operating under the mistaken expectation that Josh and Sam needed to be perfect. Because they do not have Trisomy 21, I assumed they were immune to problems. As much as it pains me to admit it, I wasn't as attentive to their needs as I should have been. I was too consumed with managing Alex's challenges.

I had to reorient myself to my role as a mother of *three*. And I'm very glad I did.

When I told people that Sam's photo was taken by the National News for a piece on Fourth of July fireworks, I realized I had not spoken my middle son's name in some time. Ditto when his team won his soccer championship and his team photo appeared on the cover of our local paper. When Josh mastered a new cello piece or created a gorgeous piece of art, I reminded myself to stop to see and hear his contributions.

If either my oldest or my middle son messed up, which they did because they are human, I found it a struggle to bite back the urge to lecture them. They deserved my patience and approval. I was doing all of us a disservice if I reserved the best of me for Alex.

Francis helped me realize that. With his guidance and encouragement, I came to understand that I want all my boys to feel a sense of belonging and inclusion, and the only way to give them that gift is by doing my best to treat them all equally while also treating them as individuals. My capacity to mother will forever be a work in progress, but part of what is involved is making the daily effort to do for all what I would do for one.

During my astrology readings, Francis told me that all children are perfect—children like Josh, Sam, and Alex. He also encouraged me to write this memoir and get my thoughts down on paper. "Don't write it for the audience; write it for yourself," he said. But before I could write the story of how Alex transformed our lives, I first had to transform myself. I had to be the mother all three of my sons deserved.

I walked into the shop I used to send birth announcements for my other two blessings feeling very different from the last times I used their services. I'd gotten over my self-consciousness about Alex's Down syndrome and had incorporated him into my life and heart with the same overwhelming and unconditional love I felt for the other two. Nevertheless, I stood, hesitant, at the counter, wondering what the solicitous sales assistant (Dienna) would think about me announcing the birth of a three-year-old toddler. The salesperson's mom, who worked in the store with her, cleared a spot at a table and brought over several huge binders of fancy announcements. Some had cute real-life photos, others adorable baby icons such as ducks, bears, or diaper pins. I chose the same ones I'd picked for Josh and Sam.

When possible, I wanted to treat Alex the same way I treated his big brothers. I'd already failed him by waiting three years to do what I should've done within three weeks of his arrival.

When Dienna asked Alex's birth weight, it saddened me that I couldn't remember.

"Let me check my orders over the years," she said. A few minutes later, she exclaimed, excitedly, "Here it is!"

The note was from January, 2008, two months after Alex's arrival. I must have thought to order the announcements, and, even though I hadn't followed through, I guessed I'd phoned the store to give them the pertinent details.

What happened? I asked myself. *Had I gotten sidetracked? Was I ashamed? Had my attention been elsewhere?*

Three years had gone by in a blur of playdates and appointments, diaper changes, feedings, bath times, walks, coffees, work, life, and family obligations.

7.9 pounds—that's how much Alex had weighed, and yet his lightness lifted my heart.

"With each child, the world begins anew," Dienna said, reminding me of the much-beloved Midrash quote we'd written on both Josh and Sam's announcements.

"Yes," I decided. "We'll go with the Midrash for Alex too."

"Do I need to include a card about why we are sending this late?" I asked Dienna.

"No!" she exclaimed. "You don't have to explain. People will understand."

I told myself not to care. People who knew us would understand. Still, I felt guilty.

Our initial shock and grief had long since been replaced. What was once "Please, G-d, don't let this be true about our baby" had turned into "Thank G-d Alex is who he is, because he's exactly who we need." Since the moment we had brought him home to us, where he belongs, Alex had been an example of love for all of us.

A baby brother for Joshua and Samuel

Alexander Gunnar לב Schwartz

October 22nd, 2008

7 pounds, 9 ounces

Named by Joshua and Samuel

"With each child the world begins anew."

- Midrash

This is the birth announcement for Alex. It was sent three years after he was born.

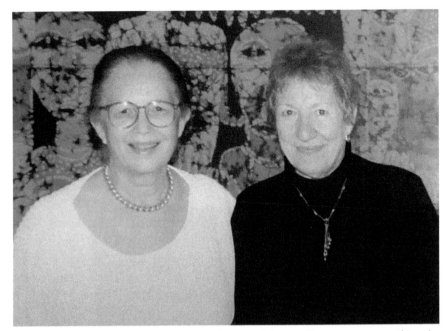

Mom, JoAnne Liebenberg Levine (right), and her college roommate/friend, Barbara Taylor Bowman. I have had the honor to communicate with Barbara these last ten years because Mom does not use a computer.

Alex was a blessing beyond measure.

When I spoke to my mother's college roommate, Barbara Bowman, she had wise words for me. "Alex is like any child. A source of joy, and pain."

The light, love, and blessings Alex brings to us cannot be put into words, although, in this book, I am attempting to do just that. The point is that we love Alex more than we can ever say. He is a lived experience that goes beyond easy articulation.

I have referred to Alex as the "architect of my soul" because he is helping to shape and mold my very essence into something more substantial. Not just me either. All of us.

If only we knew when he first arrived what we know now. Or maybe it's better that we didn't. I doubt I could have internalized and incorporated the knowledge without a direct, lived experience. We've gradually awakened to the miracle of Alex. He's a wise soul. The rest of us needed time to catch up.

In reaction to receiving Alex's baby announcement, our neighbor Ted said, "It is the thought behind the action that matters."

For the most part, I've learned not to regret the early moments in my youngest son's life. Life is a journey, and we are lucky that Alex is part of ours.

And his big brothers are an inspiration and a joy too. When Josh was in the fourth grade, he won the Kindness Award. Of all the children in his grade, my eldest son was determined to be the kindest. A year afterward, also in the fourth grade, Sam would earn the Citizen Award. I beamed with pride. I've beamed a lot over the years at the accomplishments of all my sons, but, more importantly, at their characters. I feel blessed to be raising such genuine young men.

At a baseball game during the summer of 2014, I watched my older sons, known by the rest of the spectators as "the Schwartz boys," as they played on their little league team. Although they're sixteen months apart, they were on the same team.

Alex, age six at the time, was by my side, mesmerized by his big brothers. They were quite the players. I was proud. As Alex and I, and the rest of the parents, siblings, and fans, looked on, I chatted with Colette, the very inquisitive and sweet sister of Andrew, who was on the team Josh and Sam were "versing."

That is how my son, Sam, referred to his opponents. "Mom, we're versing the other Upper Merion team this week." It still brings a smile to my face to think about his adorable and unique modes of expression.

Colette asked which foot Alex put in his mouth the most. She wanted to tickle his foot, but not if it had been in his mouth. I smiled and said it was okay to tickle his foot. Colette asked me to teach her the signs that Alex was learning so he could communicate his needs and feelings. I showed her the signs for bath, Mom, Dad, play, water, eat, thirsty, drink, shower, dog, and cat. In return, five-year-old Colette taught Alex and me Pig Latin. Evidently, her daddy, John, taught her.

Here we go, I thought. *Alex is inspiring love again.*

I could tell from his expressions that he could understand her explanations of Pig Latin. Alex is smart—a lot smarter than people might assume. He's a genius when it comes to giving and receiving love.

I often think of two quotes when thinking of all Alex has taught me:

"Remember happiness doesn't depend on who you are or what you have; it depends solely on what you think."

— Dale Carnegie

"Our soothing similarities, and delightful differences bring us together."

— MoonSong

Lessons Alex Taught Me:

- Express what is in your heart, and always be authentic.
- Don't worry what others think.
- Keep learning.
- Keep growing.
- Keep moving forward.
- Everyone can teach us something, if we remain open and curious.

Alex:

Life is an adventure. This family does not sit around. If we are not at a soccer, tennis, or baseball game, we are swimming, shopping for food, or some other activity. They like to be on the move. I do too. I love them.

4 Living

Working fulltime while raising children is a challenge. Throw in therapies, doctor visits, IEP meetings that feel like they last for days, soccer games, baseball games, tennis lessons, piano lessons, Hebrew school, swim lessons, and all the regular irregularities of raising a child with challenges, along with two other children, and trying to stay married, and it becomes near-impossible.

We have a running family joke that I like eating and Michael likes cooking, so we stay married. And Michael has been known to tell people that he hates paperwork, one of my strong suits, so that is another reason not to divorce. The truth is we love each other. Before we married, we were friends.

The rabbi who married us told us that was an auspicious foundation from which to begin a life together. "Always be friends first," he said.

Despite, or perhaps because of, our differences, Michael and I have formed an unbreakable bond. He is more stoic, less emotionally labile, and has an easier time going with the flow. He is composed during a crisis. But he is also far from one-dimensional or uptight. A person of integrity and honor, he is handsome, kind, and generous. He makes me laugh. He is smart. He also possesses artistic talent. I love collaborating with him on so much more than childrearing.

Throughout 2012, I maintained an online blog in which I wrote about my experiences mothering Alex and our other two boys. I consider that blog to have been this book's early inspiration. Michael not only supported my desire to write it, but he contributed all of the original artwork for the project. Being able to work with my husband to create something meaningful, something that reflected the creative aspects of each of us, and highlighted our unique set of skills, deepened our already strong and time-tested relationship. I can't imagine being without Michael. I am grateful for him every day.

Michael is what we in the Jewish faith refer to as a "mensch."

Caring for a child with intense and constant needs leaves little energy for relationship building. Yet, there is no one I'd rather co-parent Alex—or Josh or Sam—with than Michael. Nevertheless, as our youngest son gets older, we have come to the joint conclusion that we need more help, so we are in the process of getting a nurse forty hours per week. Having Alex with no nanny or nurse can feel overwhelming. I would not change my son for the world, but I do wish he were less afflicted by some of the tribulations that result from his Trisomy 21 diagnosis and unexplained epilepsy, which I'll write about later. So far, we've spent two years attempting to find additional at-home assistance for our family, and we still have not resolved the situation. Believe it or not, this is not unusual. There is a national nurse shortage.

At the Disabilities Law Project (now known as Disability Rights Pennsylvania), a lawyer told me more than a decade ago that the state of Pennsylvania provided several million dollars in extra funds to its HealthChoices MCOs (Managed Care Organizations), for a few years to address the nursing shortage problem. Unfortunately, that was only a partial, and temporary, fix.

The situation has been a dire disaster for years and appears to be continuing as such for families like ours. Obtaining nursing care is essential for many. Because we have a close network of family and friends, it is less essential for us, although it impacts our quality of life daily and restricts some of our choices.

While at times we are overwhelmed by caring for Alex, Josh, and Sam, Michael and I remain totally in love with all three of our boys. Dr. Cross, my obstetrician and the doctor who delivered Josh, informed me once that parents will love each child the same amount, just differently. She was right. My heart feels like it is an equilateral triangle, comprised of three direct and necessary lines. In geometry, a triangle is the strongest shape. My role as mother gives strength and substance to my life.

That said, for a long time, simply thinking about my motherly to-do list would conjure up thoughts of the 1988 movie *Women on the Verge of a Nervous Breakdown*. There were years when I wanted to hurl a blender full of gazpacho out a window while wearing coffee percolator earrings.

Good communication with my boys, my husband, and my family, was the key to getting through. I was grateful that, after taking time to reflect and process our unmet expectations, my husband was able to move forward as my true partner in life, both of us sharing feelings and coordinating logistics.

A few days after Alex was born, Michael opened up about the shock and devastation he had felt and how he had needed to shut down to assimilate the information that our youngest son was different than expected.

Three possible reactions to fear exist: fight, flight, or freeze. Michael and I were both terrified of what it would mean to have a Down syndrome son. Michael froze, whereas I swung between fight and flight, sometimes wanting to escape, and at other times feeling flooded with an inner antagonism that made me angry at the world and, truth be told, angry at my husband. Luckily, we were able to transition relatively quickly from fear to love. Not that we weren't still terrified at times, but we were less reactive. We pulled together and supported each other as we'd done for years—and will continue to do for years more.

There were and are many other supportive members of our network of allies and advocates. Alex's school team became an extension of our family. The people on his team could often be found at our home babysitting. They'd text to see how Alex was feeling when he stayed home sick. When I got breast cancer, his helper Kristen would be the one person to stay with him through my eight-hour surgery. We consider Kristen an angel on earth and one of the many miracles that would never have come into our lives without Alex. Kristen loves Alex as we do.

Having a challenged child has made me realize the truth in the old adage "It takes a village..."

Without Alex, we never would have known the love of our village. We never would have expanded our circle of support. We never would have known what was possible.

Growing up, I had the wrong perception of people with challenges, whether intellectual or physical. Before Alex, I did not understand that a challenge is not something to fear. I was ignorant. Challenges are powerful strengtheners. Challenges are opportunities to be extraordinary. My sister, Wendy, had and continues to have many challenges, including suffering from schizophrenia. I never embraced her. I wish I could have been to Wendy what Josh and Sam are to Alex. But I can't go back and rewrite the past. All I can do is love her better now. Alex opened my heart to her and to others.

Now, when I see people who use wheelchairs or oxygen or for whom life is a visible struggle, I meet their eyes, smile, and say hello.

I have begun to work more closely with the special education teacher, Karen, at the school where I teach, and we are constantly encouraging my ELL students and her to students to work together. My heart soars when my ELL students help her students in tangible, visible ways, and her students shower countless unseen blessings on my more "mainstream" student population. My experiences with Alex have made me a better teacher—a better person.

In 2011, I took a course through Temple University's Disabilities Department that exposed me to a lot of information and hands-on opportunities for learning and enlightenment. During my time at Temple, I went to visit a segregated setting for people with physical and mental disabilities. This visit reinforced my resolve.

I wanted Alex in an integrated community. Included, not separate. My third son deserves to feel he belongs. I would and will continue to do whatever I can to ensure he feels a part of life, rather than on the outside, looking in.

My other two children spoke, crawled, and walked on time. They did everything a neurologically-typical developing child does. There were scrapes and emergency room visits, some complete with ninety-mile-an-hour ambulance rides. Yet my level of worry was considerably less acute. With them, I did not have to spend five years listening to a baby monitor at night, straining to hear, and panicked that one of them would have a nocturnal seizure. (Now, after having been so limited for so long, sleep has become one of my favorite activities. Often it is polyphasic for our entire family.)

I did not have to carry Josh or Sam around the grocery store at ages three, four, five, six, seven, eight, and nine. (Thank you, again, Alex, for these strong, well-muscled arms). I did not have to plan my outings around my energy level to lift them. With Josh and Sam, we didn't invite over any creative builders or architects to see how we could keep modifying our home in ways that would allow us to effectively care for them. That's right; Alex is not just the architect of my soul; his challenges have shifted the very structure of our home as well. Or, rather, we've shifted to accommodate him. And always for the better. The process of figuring out creative ways to ensure that Alex's needs are met and that our family can continue to function well as a unit and individually has made each of us more innovative and adaptable.

But there is always that ever-present sense of worry, which was even more intense when Alex was younger. I never knew that level of worry with Josh or Sam.

Every bite of food they took did not have to be policed as a potential choking hazard. I did not have to search my brain—one not skewed toward the domestic that has always hated cooking—for what I might feed them that would not trigger a seizure. No notebooks were kept on when they awoke at night, how they eliminated, or what they ate that day.

I did not correct strangers when they used the R word. I myself used it. While I thought I was open to differences, I was by no means as open then as I am now that Alex is here.

I did not understand the pain generated each time the R word is spoken. Since Alex, I have pledged never to use it.

Every once in a while, someone will see me with Alex and say, "He's lucky to have you." But that's not how I feel at all. We're lucky to have him.

My eldest sons have evolved into people with empathy and compassion for everyone they meet. They grew up hearing Michael and me espouse a "spread the word to end the word" philosophy. When Josh and Sam were still in elementary school, Josh came home one day and informed us that he had overheard a little girl in Sam's class call a boy (another student in the class) "retarded."

Josh told the girl, "My baby brother has the same thing. He is not the R-word. He is just my brother."

She replied, "So?"

He walked away.

Sam heard this and said, "I would have yelled at her."

I explained that it was wonderful for both of them to champion those with challenges, and I gently encouraged Sam to remember that the only way to dissipate hatred is with love. Some people aren't lucky enough to know what we knew, but we can plant the seeds of knowledge, then go on with our lives while hoping the seeds we planted might take root.

I see the potential in people like Alex. Anything is possible. I did not understand any of this before.

George, Grace's son, has continued to provide an enduring example of hope to our family. He is nineteen now. I still get a yearly Christmas card from him. Each one is a reminder never to underestimate children with challenges. I hope my own son may one day embark on a large and unlimited life, following in the footsteps of those who have gone before.

In her book *Seeing Trees*, Nancy Ross Hugo explains how when those prickly round ball things that dangle off trees fall to the ground, we are all so annoyed by them. What we don't see is that inside each prickly ball lies many seeds with unlimited potential to grow.

I potty-trained our other boys, and they went effortlessly on their own. Alex is potty-trained, but for years he could not tell us when he had to go. We had to anticipate his needs. Eventually, we were able to teach him a sign for bathroom. But it took time, patience, and more than a few "whoopsies!" I had it easy with Josh and Sam and did not realize it. Alex is harder. He depends on us both to respect his need for autonomy and to know when he has to have help. This difficulty is rewarding in ways I will never be able to fully express. Parenting Alex feels as nuanced and beautiful as a dance. Sometimes, he leads and I follow. Other times, the sequence is reversed. But we are in constant flow, and he exhibits more grace and enriches my life more than I ever imagined possible.

The therapies (speech, occupational therapy, physical therapy, and special education) Alex receives help him beyond any hopes we had when he first began incorporating these modalities into his life.

Alex started occupational therapy when he was only three days old. He was still in the NICU, hooked up to monitors. The therapist came in and worked with him there. I will forever be grateful for the forward-thinking hospital staff. I was much too shell-shocked to think about the logistics of my newborn boy's later life and functioning, but they knew early intervention was essential, so they got Alex the help he needed.

Not that I didn't have my own help to offer.

Marie Weiss, a mom from Wayne Elementary School where I worked, told me shortly after Alex was born that "A hug is the best therapy." I have to agree. Love and hugs seem to help Alex more than any other treatment or therapy. This is not a problem for me. I have an unlimited supply, and I gladly give them to all my sons.

I think having Alex made me realize just how much we could all use affection. He needs lots of peace and love. He cannot stand anger or stress. I see in his little body the impact negative emotions have on him. I know many people suffer from exposure to painful feelings, but Alex's sensitivity has heightened my awareness and vigilance. Now, I make more of a concerted effort to keep things tranquil, and we've all reaped the rewards. Peaceful does not mean boring.

Through Alex, I have met play-writers, actors, authors, ballerinas, notables such as Jill Biden and Senator Daylin Leach, and others who may not be widely known but are nevertheless incredible in their own ways. Moms and children whose lives are a mirror image of Alex and me, people who help me walk this path of a life that may be touched by Down syndrome but is only elevated because of that. An up, not down, life.

Alex has been my guide. Through his daily struggles and successes, he reminds me that something wonderful is always about to happen. The only limits are the ones we set for ourselves.

Part of this book was first included in a play called *A Fierce Kind of Love*, written by Suli Holum and directed by David Bradley. Holum and Bradley interviewed me in a number of what they referred to as "listening sessions." They asked me to share my experiences raising Alex, and they incorporated some of what I told them into their creative vision. The play draws on the experiences of many generations of parents like me—mothers and fathers with children whose lives have been marked by challenges. An excerpt of my book was read on stage by the actor Lee Ann Etzold as well as on Dan Gottlieb's popular National Public Radio (NPR) show, *Voices in the Family*. I was driving up to work at Radnor Elementary when the show came on the radio. Even though I should've gone into the building to prepare for my workday and the impending influx of students, my principal, Terry, had already given me permission to come in late so I could finish listening. I will never forget how I heard my words through Lee Ann Etzold, and thought how many other people were able to hear them through this program. I hope my words touched others even just a fraction of how much Alex's nonverbal communication touches those he encounters.

I was fortunate to see *A Fierce Kind of Love* performed. It included actors with disabilities. As I watched, my eyes filled with tears of gratitude. Not only was the play about overcoming adversity and loving with open arms and an expansive heart, but it was an act of love, inviting differently abled people to embrace their skillsets and shine their spotlights on those of us lucky enough to be seated in the audience. After seeing it once, I wasn't done. I had to see it again, to soak in every word and feeling.

The next time I went, I brought my friend, Sara Byala, with me. Sara is the friend who took my dreams and prayers to the wall in Israel (the Kotel) when she watched her son become a Bar Mitzvah there. A Bar Mitzvah is when a boy becomes a man in the Jewish religion. There is a special service, and usually a party. Sara snapped a photo of my yellow Post-it notes with my prayers on them. This is the kind of friend she is—extraordinary. We exercise together with

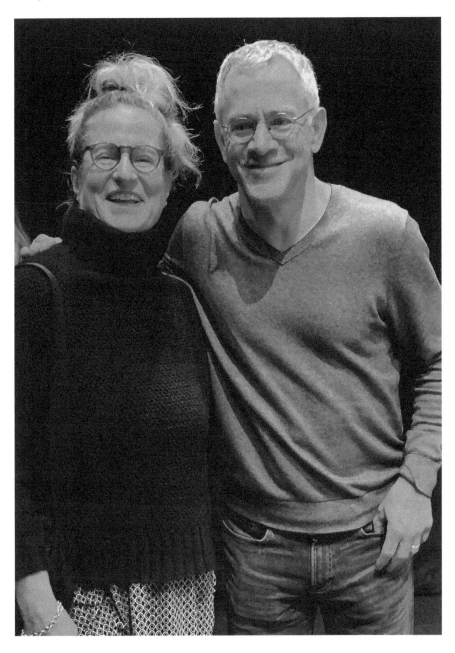

Me and the director, David Bradley, at the performance of *A Fierce Kind of Love*. I have been fortunate to see the play three times.

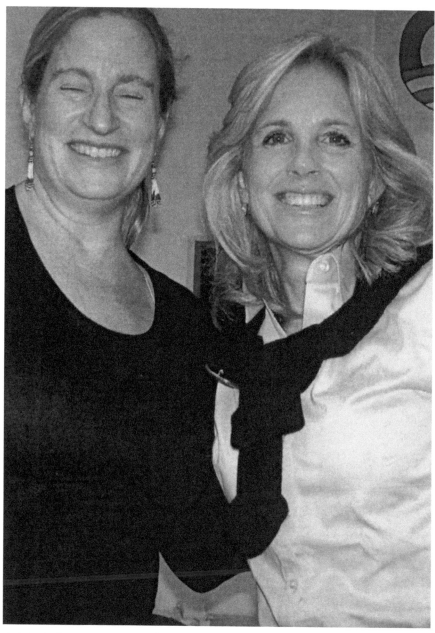

Right before President Obama was elected, when I was pregnant with Alex,
I met Jill Biden at a local event in Upper Merion, Pennsylvania

our Tribe (main line fitness group) three times a week. She encourages me mentally, physically, and spiritually, and my life is enriched because of her solicitude and the solidarity we share. Having Sara at my side made my second experience viewing the play even richer than the first.

I knew I would never forget the play. Each performance made an indelible imprint on my heart. *A Fierce Kind of Love* will continue to be performed, forever memorializing my and others' experiences in the hearts and minds of anyone lucky enough to see it. I was asked to continue to participate in future listening sessions and to bring along my entire book to share. I'm grateful that this book has now become a reality. Perhaps, it will inspire more life-affirming works of art. Alex has taught me the value of collaborative creativity.

Funnily enough, before I ever knew how Alex would be a special light in my life, his spirit was working within me to bring extraordinary experiences my way. When I was still pregnant with Alex, I met Jill Biden at an event in King of Prussia (Upper Merion Township). I was there with my neighbor, Carol Flannery.

And, as you can see, Alex attended too. He was in my belly.

President Obama would be president the year Alex was born. I got to email his highest advisor's mom, Barbara Bowman: Hallelujah! My mom was her friend and college roommate. Because my mom did not know how to use a computer, I was blessed to be enlisted as her email ally. I have sent numerous emails to Barbara Bowman on behalf of my technologically-challenged mother and, in the process, Barbara and I have developed a friendship of our own. Barbara's wisdom and light come through with each of her emails.

I met a fellow mom, Paige Figi, through Facebook. I often consult her when I need help figuring out some aspect of Alex's care. Paige is exceptional and a true pioneer when it comes to advocating for challenged children's rights. Paige's story can be found in the CNN story "Weed" (https://tinyurl.com/gupta-weed). Her experiences inspired me to do research into alternative and nontraditional treatment interventions and explore every possible option for helping Alex be healthier and happier.

Brenda Dixon-Gottschild is a professor, dancer, and writer. I met her through Facebook as well, and, after having the extraordinary opportunity of seeing her dance with Ballet X, I met her after the performance, along with her husband Helmut. Brenda makes positive, uplifting comments on my wall about Alex. She brings the same grace with which she dances to her interactions, and I feel blessed to have her in my life.

All these people, and so many more, have demonstrated the need for inclusion and incorporation of everyone. Their tolerance, love, and acceptance reverberate through me as I reflect on my own inner evolution to develop a more expansive attitude.

I was parented to appreciate differences—to accept all. I had playdates with all kinds of children when I was young. I was taken to the Philadelphia Art Museum, sometimes against my wishes. People, art, and books were held in high esteem in my home. My mom and dad showed me that what matters most is how we treat others. Whenever I was with my mom in public, I could expect to have many conversations with strangers, who, after a few minutes with her, became friends. Some even ended up hugging her!

Once when I was driving with Mom, at a stoplight, she got out to say hello to another driver because she had a license plate from her beloved Minnesota. I was mortified. And, yet, I believe my mother's attitude secretly infiltrated my spirit.

Later, as an adult, I would approach a fellow mom, Kate Sanderson, at the Wayne Elementary School where I taught because her license had Minnesota on it. I talked to her, just like I'd seen Mom do while I slumped down in my seat, rolling my eyes and praying for a less embarrassing mother. It turned out that Kate was all too happy to chat about Minnesota. She was glad I approached her and grateful for the opportunity to reminisce. Not only that—Kate knew about my grandpa, Jack Liebenberg.

"You're related to him!" she exclaimed. "He designed two hundred movies theaters, churches, and synagogues. He's a legend in Minneapolis."

I had the example of two parents who were open and receptive to connecting with others' hearts, but it took my youngest son to crack my shell and make me willing to embody the example I grew up with.

My dad kept stickers of every country's flag on his car bumper. People from every country held a place in his heart. His friend, Larry Buchsbaum, according to his three daughters, spoke eleven different languages and survived the Holocaust. Having himself fought in World War II, Dad earned a silver star for his bravery and valor under pressure. Not just bravery and valor—bravado. He had to pretend he had bullets in an empty gun to stave off an enemy attack. Dad was in awe of Larry Buchsbaum. I was in awe of Dad. He was brave. He was also cultured and sophisticated. He blessed us all with his love of literature and writing. During one of the last visits I had with Dad, at our home, he brought peach, perfume-scented roses.

Mom and Dad divorced when I was ten. I was jealous that, when they were my age, my sisters, Susie and Wendy, were able to experience life with our parents together. It was hard. A wise psychologist in the child guidance department at CHOP (Children's Hospital of Philadelphia), told my mom, "You only get one dad and one mom."

My parents tried to honor their roles, as well as each other, even though they ended their romantic relationship. The way they were with each other offered a lesson in love for me. I'm sure a lot of pain led to their decision to separate, but they never inflicted that pain on us. They were kind and gentle, put our needs ahead of theirs, and did what they could to ensure we didn't suffer as a result of their split. Nevertheless, I wanted a family where everyone stayed together. It's funny because I wanted the family I now have. And I'm not so sure my own nuclear family unit would be as unbreakably bonded as we are without Alex to act as an adhesive.

Nevertheless, both my parents taught me that positivity feeds the soul. Even so, I think part of me did not always fully embrace differences.

I struggled with fear of the unknown as well as internalized social norms and standards that I now realize didn't serve me. Our society values intelligence, beauty, and physical strength. Sometimes, in doing so to the exclusion of other noble attributes, we miss seeing the emotional intelligence and other gifts we all have the capacity to share. Now I see how valuable people of all abilities and challenges are. Alex taught me this.

Alex is a gift beyond measure. He attends public school. It was not easy at first. I can still remember his first Individualized Education Program (IEP) meeting. During these meetings, a team made up of parents or caregivers, teachers, and therapists, makes a plan to help a child acquire the lessons needed in a way they can digest and assimilate. Each individual student receives a tailored approach to education that honors their limitations and embraces their strengths. This collaborative process for designing an individualized curriculum is essential for integrating differently-abled students into more mainstream environments. Once a plan is agreed upon, an official document is created to reflect the decisions the IEP team has made. The plan can later be modified based on outcomes, changes in skills and circumstances, and a host of other variables. It is tailored to each child's needs. I cannot overstate the value of the IEP's emphasis on teamwork.

For Alex and other such challenged children, there are many, many adults who interact with them on a daily basis and see them function in different contexts. Having different perspectives is helpful.

Even though I've worked in education most of my professional life and was in the field long before having Alex, I never fully appreciated the value of an IEP until my third son entered the educational system. Under the law, every child is entitled to FAPE (free appropriate public education). They are also entitled to LRE (a least restrictive environment), a protected right of every child and the public education system's responsibility.

IDEA (The Individuals with Disabilities Education Act) is a four-part piece of American legislation that ensures students with a disability are provided with FAPE tailored to their needs.

Surrounded by a whole lot of serious faces, I felt awkward and unsure. Luckily for me (or so I thought), I'd brought not just our advocate but Jessica Gold. Jessica is an incredibly talented lawyer who won the Gaskin case. According to the Public Interest Law Center, the Gaskin case resulted from the following:

> In the early 1990s, Pennsylvania had the second worst rate of inclusion of students with disabilities in regular education classrooms in the country. And, when students were included, it was often without meaningful support. Few regular education teachers had any training in teaching students with disabilities, and schools were often unwilling to provide needed resources. Although the law places responsibility for compliance with IDEA on the state, Pennsylvania did little to make sure its districts were actually complying with the law. And, when it became clear they were failing, the state did little to fix the problem.
>
> We filed the lawsuit Gaskin v. Commonwealth on June 30, 1994, seeking to increase the number of children with disabilities educated with their non-disabled peers, and to make sure inclusion would work as required by IDEA. To reach those goals, the lawsuit sought to change Pennsylvania's systems for training districts in inclusion, and for monitoring, and enforcing their compliance. The suit was filed on behalf of a class of 280,000 special education

students, twelve named plaintiffs, and eleven disabilities advocacy organizations.[1]

While the initiatives that arose out of this landmark case have helped, we still have a long way to go to improve our educational system and make it more accessible for children with challenges. But I didn't know what to expect as I walked into the room for my first IEP meeting.

I had Jessica by my side.

I quickly discovered I wasn't lucky at all.

As soon as we walked in, Jessica, my lawyer, was thrown out of the meeting. We had not asked in advance if she could be present. We didn't know we needed to. I wanted Jessica in the meeting with us. I wanted someone with experience dealing with and understanding children such as Alex and families like ours by my side. We'd discussed Michael and my feelings, wants, and needs for our son. And although I've always been a dedicated advocate for all my children, I was far from familiar with the way the system worked. My role as an educator hadn't prepared me. After all, although I am a dedicated teacher, love my students, and like to think I treat them as if they were my own, I am able to maintain greater perspective and distance than when dealing with a situation that I know could impact any of my three sons' happiness.

Jessica would fight to have Alex included no matter what. And not just brought into the classroom on special days. I wanted my son to be a full citizen of the school. A boy like any other, with friends and homework.

It turned out that even without Jessica in the room, I was able to articulate my desires for my youngest.

"I want him included 100 percent of the time." I was adamant, if misinformed.

The team members explained they thought Alex should be incorporated into the more mainstream environment 50 percent of the time. My son needed space to process and work independently, they argued. Full inclusion would be too much. I left angry and discouraged, but I've since come to realize we all want what's best for Alex. He is happy—thriving. And he feels included even if he does require space and time to address his unique needs with the support and love of a more individualized approach.

---

[1] https://www.pubintlaw.org/cases-and-projects/gaskin-v-commonwealth/

We have come a long way since that day with Jessica Gold by my side. Alex is included 50 percent logistically, but with 100 percent love. He is able to spend his days in the classroom with an aide to assist his teacher in targeting things he needs help with, such as eating, using the potty, learning, and playing.

He is happy. He is also surrounded by a community of friends. Upon seeing him, the other kids in his class scream, "Alex!"

Over the years of experiencing people interacting with Alex, I've come to realize that it often takes less time for children to intuit what is harder for adults to realize. Children who need assistance can possess a special kind of spirit-energy that is a blessing and joy to be around. Alex's classmates know what I know. Alex may not be able to communicate in the same way as his peers, yet he is there, fully and completely aware, and with a capacity for connection I can only aspire to. My third son is a whole individual. He is not less than anyone else, and his contributions are not less valuable merely because they are different.

Alex has become a valued member of his community of learners. He is a friend and a boy like any other, who simply needs assistance with some tasks that come easily to others his age.

Alex's teacher, Mrs. Kim Gambone, is a gift. She informs us daily about Alex's struggles and successes. She maintains a written notebook with details about his progress and his activities and, as if that weren't enough, composes a multi-paragraph daily email to let Michael and me know how Alex's day was. Lately, she has been taking a photo and adding it to her text-update. She explains the intricacies of his health challenges. She helps me fill out the millions of forms that raising a child in the special education system requires. Kim Gambone is an angel. We are thankful that Alex has her as a teacher. And she, in turn, reminds us daily that she is thankful for the value Alex adds to her life.

As part of the daily recap, Kim allows Alex to communicate directly with us about his day by taking the time to ask him about things and remaining with him while he touches the card on his iPad to communicate his thoughts and feelings for himself. It's important that, just because our son is not yet verbal, he never feels he doesn't have a voice.

From parenting Alex, I've learned that people sometimes see a limitation and get stuck within a narrow focus of what that means, placing unfair restrictions on the person who, although challenged, is capable of so much more than others assume. Today, when I tell people about Alex, I will usually say he has Trisomy 21 because people don't know what that means. Then they don't bring a host of misconceptions to the situation. I also have chosen to use phrases like "challenged" or "differently abled," as opposed to "disabled." I don't want to perpetuate the cultural misbelief that Down syndrome has to be a "downer." Alex has elevated our entire world, and I want others to know that.

When people ask me about Alex's progress, or lack thereof, and point out all the things he cannot do, I smile and say, "Not yet." Alex can't walk yet, talk yet, live an unassisted life yet. But there are no limits to what might be possible in the future. In the meantime, I try to remember to rejoice in the process. The small moments. The victories along the way. And not just in Alex's life, but in my own life as well. If I go for a run and am able to get just a little farther than expected, or if Michael and I share an especially tender moment, or Josh or Sam has a great day, I take the time to savor that. Before Alex, everything seemed to be about the destination. Now, my son who can't yet dance has taught me to dance through life's daily miracles.

Alex's school nurse, Barbara Dale, is another incredible person. We speak daily to keep Alex happy and healthy. In case Alex has had a seizure at school, or at home, we need to communicate about that and come up with a strategy for supporting him in meeting any needs that may arise from a change in his situation. Sometimes, we have to tweak his schedule, giving him time for an extra nap, providing a snack, or reworking his calendar so he can skip a therapy and give his brain and body an opportunity to rebalance.

Sure, with Alex, I have had to be much more hands-on than with the other two, but in that process, I have cultivated more gratitude than I ever would have believed possible. (I thought of myself as grateful before. Little did I know....)

We are full of blessings. Alex's daily angels are a huge reason why.

At a recent haircut appointment, as soon as Alex and I entered the salon, a little boy yelled, "Alex!"

While at the University of Pennsylvania for an ELL conference (I was attending for work and not in my capacity as the mother of a challenged child), Susan, the assistant superintendent of Alex's district was there. When she found out I was Alex's mom, she said to give him a hug! How lucky to have a celebrity son, a boy people love for his purity, sacred spirit, and capacity to give and receive love.

Our friend Beth told me that "Alex's laugh is pretty much all you need."

Another beautiful friend, Jessica Sontag, said, "He is a gift."

And he is. There is a quote from Jessica's dad that resonates deep within me whenever I think about how Alex has exceeded all my expectations and added daily value to my life: "It's only as hard as we make it."

Lessons Alex Taught Me:

- Having a purpose and doing meaningful work have the capacity to make life beautiful.

- Using our knowledge to help others feeds our souls as well as theirs.

- If you are neuro-typical, it does not mean your achievements are better than those of someone who is not.

- Inclusion does not only happen in the classroom. It happens in the playground, in the hallway, at the lunch table, in the swimming pool, at birthday parties, during school board meetings, at staff meetings, and in the community.

- Our light gives light to others.

- Hugs are the best therapy.

- We can be stronger and do more together.

- There is no I in TEAM.

- When you think one thing is a certain way, look underneath to unearth its true potential.

- ANYTHING IS POSSIBLE.

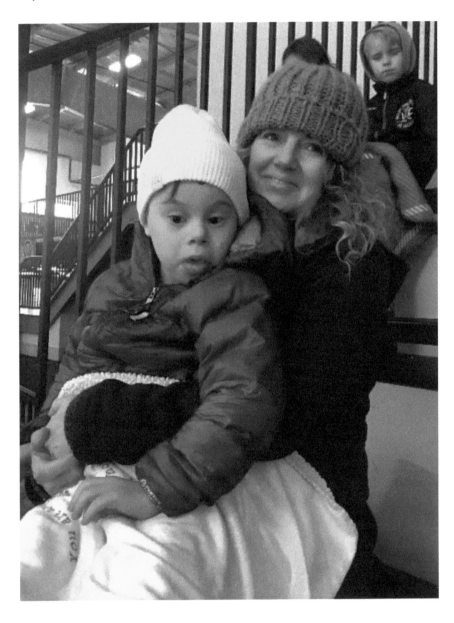

Alex stayed with Jessica Lowenadler Sontag and her family, while Michael and I had some time away. Alex loved watching her son, Jonas's hockey game, and being with her other children, Anders and Mia.

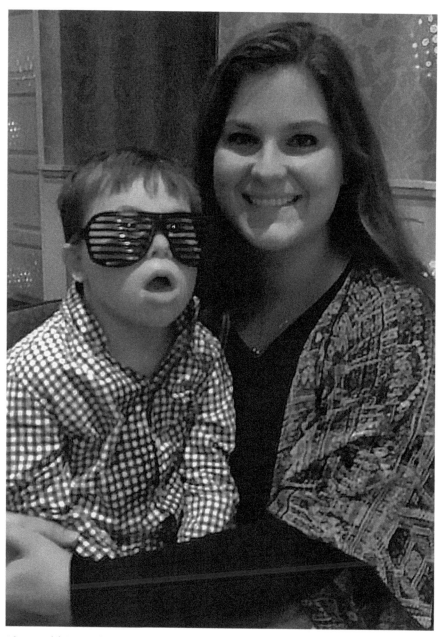

Alex and his teacher/helper Kristen. Kristen loves, and cares for Alex as if he were part of her family.

Alex:

Mrs. Callahan, my third grade teacher, is putting Go Noodle on the smartboard. I cannot wait! Look at my friends; they are jumping in the air. I would love to jump high. Hands are flying in a dance with their feet. I can't wait to dance too. My helper is pushing my chair to the side of my friends in the front of the room. Yay! I am grooving out too. My feet are flying up from my chair. My body is going back and forth in time to the music video. I love to be included. This is fun! I am happiest with my friends.

5   **Bumps**

"The Uninvited Guest" by Nancy Schwartz

Y*ou come without warning or invitation. Jolting us from our slumber with your horror. The terror spreads across our baby's face. His face contorts in a mix of fear and confusion. Sometimes his face is stretched wide like a silent scream. More often you make our boy cry out loud, and you jerk him around as if you are a bully in the schoolyard. Stealing our precious sleep. But not our hope. Not our resolve. All is well. You may be stealthy and quiet. Or loud and mean.... But we are stronger. We have love, faith, and hope. All is well.*

Alex had a fever that day. He tried to sleep, and finally the Tylenol worked its magic. He was sleeping in my arms. As I cradled him, I felt a shake like an earthquake. Unknown to me, the earthquake was a grand mal seizure. His entire body shook. His mouth contorted, and his eyes blinked. Shockwaves rippled through his little body.

I woke Michael. "Michael, I think something is wrong with Alex."

"You are nuts," he said—his standard, lighthearted response to what he assumed was yet another overreaction from me.

It's true that I can sometimes be overly attentive to the point where I imagine problems that aren't there, whereas my husband is laidback and sometimes minimizes things that do actually require attention. On the whole, we balance each other out.

This time, though, I knew something was wrong. I felt it. Michael went back to sleep, and I sat awake, long into the night, bracing myself for another earthquake.

It didn't come immediately, but it did come, and when it did, it shook us all.

We were visiting my mom in Surf City, Long Beach Island. Sleeping arrangements were less than desirable. Our entire family was relegated to the floor.

The next night, Alex drifted off to sleep between Michael and me, both of us reaching out a hand to hold him as he headed off into the oblivion of sleep. I was glad Michael was touching him too.

This time, when the earthquake hit, he felt it as well.

"That's weird," he said.

Panicked, I phone the doctor.

"Sounds like a fever-induced seizure," Dr. Robinson tried to assure me long distance.

Later, we would have an EEG and scans of Alex's brain. Dr. Dan Long, a neurologist at Children's Hospital of Philadelphia (CHOP), explained there was no reason for the seizures. "They just are," he said, leaving me both grateful for his honesty and annoyed by my perception of the medical community's incompetence. Okay, they weren't incompetent, but I wanted answers and all we were left with were questions.

The doctor told me to look at it differently. "It's good you don't have a reason," he explained. "Unexplained epilepsy is a better alternative than a brain tumor or another diagnosis."

This was scarier than hearing Alex had Down syndrome.

Down syndrome I knew, or at least had a mild familiarity with. I knew students, other kids, people living with intellectual challenges....

Epilepsy (what it's called when a person has more than one seizure) I didn't know. Medicine was prescribed. Adding Trileptal to Alex's daily routine felt like a disaster. It made our already challenged child seem out of it. He was unhappy. He cried often. My heart ached with helplessness. Alex needed medication to prevent against seizures, but the medication was making him not himself anymore.

One day at work, I got a call from his teacher. "Alex is drooling in red. He is unresponsive."

My heart dropped. My son was bleeding. He was sick.

His dose of Trileptal had just been increased by his newest neurologist. We have had six different neurologists. This latest doctor's hope was to let our son eat a cupcake (glucose can be a trigger for epileptic episodes) and not have a seizure. I could not breathe.

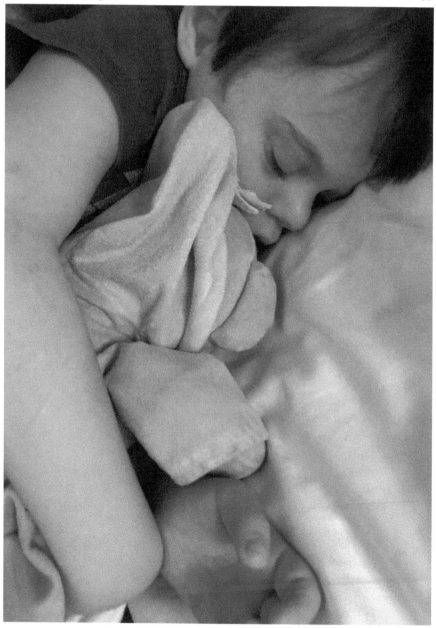

Alex snuggles the bear Sam gave him. Bear has been there for Sam from the time he was a baby. This is one of the most generous heart gifts Alex has ever received.

As I struggled to comprehend the news that Alex was drooling blood, I remembered when my dad was alive. "Keep the faith," he would remind us. Like that day in the NICU three years previously, when I wanted to make Alex breathe, I wanted to take his seizures away. I had no control then, or now. Faith in the face of fear is how we can cope with the unimaginable situations that can occur with any child, and often with children who have medical challenges.

Alex is sensitive to medicine. The increased dosage nearly took his precious life. He was not moving or breathing well. Rushing to drive to his school, my mind raced, and thought of all we could lose. I could barely concentrate on my driving. Michael met me at Saint David's Nursery School. We got him evaluated at the emergency room. Thankfully, this incident is a memory, and not the moment we lost him. But I still carry the weight of worry for his safety and wellbeing. I learned from this episode how doctors need to know about his vulnerability toward medication.

It wasn't the doctor's fault. It wasn't the medicine. It was the combination of chemicals and Alex's delicate system.

A new neurologist prescribed a new medicine, Depakote, then Onfi. These are strong chemical compounds that again incited that scary zombie look in my beautiful young son. Easy laughter and bright, contagious smiles became almost nonexistent. It was a very hard time. I did not know what to do. I wanted Alex to be a *threenager*. A three-year-old with only fun on his agenda, not neurologist appointments and medication-induced fogginess. Sure, he wasn't walking or talking yet, but his Down syndrome never made him unable to participate in the abundance of life. Now, this. Lamictal. Another seizure medicine. More appointments. More tests.

It was all so unfair.

I do not watch television. After Seinfeld ended, I didn't see a reason to. Therefore, it was unusual that I was in front of the TV, CNN on in the background, when a story called "Weed" came on. I thank G-D that I happened to hear that story that day.

Immediately, I became glued to the television as I watched Charlotte Figi's petite body shake as our Alex did. I could not believe my ears or my eyes. Here was this beautiful little girl, Charlotte, having many seizures, and not able to eat, walk, or exist as a happy, healthy child.

That was when I first heard about Charlotte's Web. No, not the well-known children's book. Charlotte's Web was the name of the medicine in the CNN story. This life-improving, soul-sustaining oil was named for Charlotte Figi, the little girl it helped save.

When the Figi family tried this medicine made by the Stanley Brothers, miraculously, Charlotte became seizure-free, walking, dancing, and living. A high quality of life, not merely existing. I knew Alex's seizures were mild in amount and length compared to Charlotte's. Something about the way her body shook like his and how this magic oil took away her seizures made me stop.

Through Facebook, I friended Paige Figi, Charlotte's mom. I reached out to her to express my gratitude for her experience and tell her a bit about Alex. I could not believe how generous she was with her time. Paige agreed to speak to me on the phone. What a blessing!

I can still conjure up the memory of her voice.

"I know this works," she told me. "You could be the first mom to give this oil to your son with Down syndrome."

Thanks to Paige, I was able to arrange a phone consultation with Charlotte's doctor in Colorado.

"Yes," the doctor told me, "this could help your son."

Over the years, I would stay in touch with Paige. Through her, I would be exposed to countless other avenues of exploration, receiving answers to the questions I'd been harboring and finding at least partial solutions to seemingly unsolvable problems.

Eventually, I would get support from Realm of Caring (ROC), a not-for-profit organization. It provides support services for hospitals, doctors, parents, caregivers, and researchers. ROC stays at the front of cannabis science. It tries to find the best treatments and applications for cannabinoid therapies. They offer education, advocacy, and a digital research library. I am able to call or email them with questions. This is life-changing support. This organization has helped me to get a handle on Alex's seizures. By registering Alex's diagnosis with them, we qualified for a discounted price on Charlotte's Web oil.

Some of the CHOP doctors thought I was crazy. They did not think marijuana oil would work for Alex. I tried to explain that the oil is actually considered hemp. It could be purchased at Whole Foods in other forms.

The word *marijuana* is a combination of the name Mary and Juan. Today, the term denotes an illegal, recreational drug. Referring to a potentially life-saving tool in the same way as a teenage party-drug undermines our ability to critically examine its efficacy as a potential tool for treating illness. The true term is cannabis.

Thanks to the efforts of many moms, like Lolly Bentch, and dads in Pennsylvania, the state in which my family lives became the twenty-fourth state to legalize medical marijuana. If you're not familiar with cannabis advocacy, which most people are not, Lolly Bentch is a pivotal figure. According to literature put out by the Pennsylvania Medical Cannabis Society, "Lolly Bentch was a founding member of Campaign for Compassion, a group of mothers who had faith that their children, many with intractable epilepsy, would benefit from marijuana products. Campaign for Compassion aggressively lobbied legislators to pass S.B.3, the state's medical cannabis bill. Governor Tom Wolf signed it into law on April 17, 2016. Lolly now serves as the patient liaison for the Department of Health's Cannabis Service. Lolly has an eight-year-old autistic daughter who suffers from hundreds of seizures each day. As a patient liaison, Bentch's job is to ensure patients, caregivers, and advocates are represented as the medical marijuana program takes shape. Health Department spokeswoman April Hutcheson said, "Bentch's unique experience gives her the perfect background to make sure the voices of our parents, and caregivers are heard."

Many political influencers can be credited with helping bring these life-giving products into the public awareness and legalizing their usage. The efforts that Senators Daylin Leach and Mike Folmer and their teams have made have provided Michael and me with the tools to help our child. Daylin even helped erase the stigma around this medicine. He traveled to Colorado where he conducted on-the-ground research into how they used the programs there to help patients. Then, upon his return, Daylin created an initiative that could allow people across Pennsylvania to come together and learn about cannabis. I was able to attend these teachings at Saint Joseph's University with Lolly Bentch and many others. Lolly is amazing. I am blessed to call her my friend. And the entire family is thankful for her assistance. Even with the help of friends, advocates, and political figures, obtaining the medical marijuana card for Alex was a process. It should be easier. Parents should be able to get these herbal medicines with the same ease with which they obtain synthetic meds.

People need CBD. Some need THC (tetrahydrocannabinol), one of at least 113 cannabinoids identified in cannabis. THC is the principal psychoactive constituent of cannabis. The term THC also refers to cannabinoid isomers. Our own brains make this substance.

Some need THCA. Tetrahydro-cannabinoid acid is the non-psychoactive precursor of the primary active constituent of marijuana, cannabis sativa.

Admittedly, cannabis is not for everyone. But it is a medicine so it should be accessible to anyone it can help, regardless of age or condition.

Alex has used the Charlotte's Web oil for more than three years now. His newest and greatest neurologist, Dr. April Ray, at CHOP helped us wean Alex from the drugs that did not help him. She has been our advocate and ally in helping to give our third son the quality of life we aspire to help all our boys attain. I won't go into a digression here about insurance and the medical system at large; however, I should mention that we refused to use Alex's secondary insurance because it would have forced him to see a different doctor than the one we determined was best qualified to take care of him. We want Alex to have the best medical doctors we can find, and we want to optimize his chances of thriving in a world not yet equipped to empower challenged children.

While on Charlotte's Web oil, Alex gained weight for the first time in three years. He is getting taller, seemingly by the week. Alex's ability to make and hold eye contact has improved, as has his capacity for continued engagement. He is also more focused and happier. Charlotte's Web is well worth every penny. This medicine is not free. We make sacrifices to afford it. We may not travel to exotic places or throw fancy parties, but Michael and I love and care for all of our boys.

Josh, Sam, and Alex are all happier now that Alex can use Charlotte's Web oil. It was worrisome for all of us to see Alex's light dimmed by the aggressive medical interventions, and we missed his radiance. Now, once again, we hear his laughter and see his gorgeous smile. It has not been easy to find his sweet spot. I have had many talks with the amazing team at Realm of Caring. One mom, Meagan, advised, "When you start to see daytime seizures, do a reboot."

A reboot is when the child comes off all oil for a day, and we start small with teensy dosing to see what the perfect amount for seizure control is. The neurologist was able to access information from the Realm of Caring. They have a digital library and lots of information to help educate on this medicine. After the reboot, we were once again able to lower his dosage.

Decreasing his dose of Charlotte's Web oil helped a ton since he is so sensitive. A fellow mom at Realm of Caring explained that she

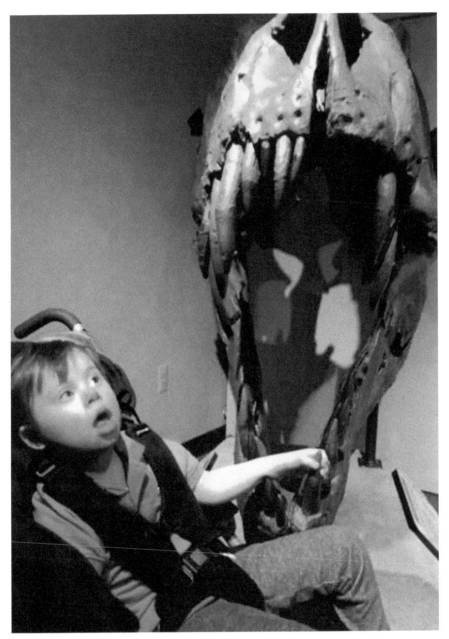

Alex had a field trip to the Museum of Natural History in Philadelphia. He was testing the dental care of this dinosaur.

kept a notebook to keep track of her child's symptoms, habits, reactions, schedule, and needs. Getting relief from these seizures is a dance. Sometimes, the traditional medicine needs changes, or Alex's CW oil amounts need to be tweaked. When he is undergoing a growth spurt, seizure activity can increase, thus prompting us to revisit his current dosages and revise our existing treatment protocol.

As I listened to this mother talk about the value of her symptom-management recordkeeping, I thought, *I should do the same.*

She agreed.

"Write down when he wakes up, or if he has trouble sleeping at night," she counseled. "Write what he eats. Write when he has a seizure. When he eliminates. How the elimination seems. Explain in your notebook how the seizure looks."

She told me she had noticed in her own daughter that being constipated could cause a seizure.

"Try and keep his diet healthy," she advised. "See what works and what doesn't."

I acted like a scientist. I wrote everything down. I looked for patterns, triggers that seemed to cause seizures.

Our CHOP neurologist, Dr. Ray, said we should focus on the big picture. Were the seizures better or worse over time? She still recommended using pharmaceutical drugs if we were seeing more seizures. But she supported our decision when we held to our faith that the oil could work. Her support was instrumental. We have never felt more confident in the non-traditional interventions we have tried with Alex.

I noted detail after detail in my notebook and, before long, I'd made connections I hadn't been aware of before. White sugar, and sometimes white flour, caused seizures for Alex, as did chemicals, dyes, or overly-processed food. I have since eliminated white sugar and white flour from Alex's diet. The family as a whole tries to eat healthily, not only in support of Alex but because it is good to avoid refined foods. We are far from perfect, however. I attribute this to the fact that we don't have the same incentive as Alex. Plus, because we can procure our own food and Alex can't (yet), we don't have anyone overseeing our choices.

Alex's neurologist agreed that some of her patients with seizure disorders are glucose intolerant. I noted that when Alex is sick, stressed, or overtired, he is more susceptible to episodes. He needs exercise, and since he does not walk—yet—swimming has become his sport. Alex swims with the swim team members at Bryn Mawr

College and with his dad at our family gym, Lifetime. Lately, we've been lowering his already teensy dose of Depakote to see if that helps him. It seems to, although it may still be too early to tell. We are also now trying to find the right combination of alternative oils. It is an ever-moving target.

Currently, it seems as if Charlotte's Web in the morning and Haleigh's Hope in the evening helps Alex to exist within his sweet spot.

Jasmin at Realm of Caring helped me understand that using CW oil at a good dose for Alex in addition to rubbing some CBD[2] oil on his feet could help. I have purchased Haleigh's Hope, 20:1 and 15:1, and have tried that on his feet at night in addition to his daily oral dose of Charlotte's Web oil. The ratios stand for the amount of CBD to THC. The HH (Haleigh's Hope) that is 15:1 is the one that seems to be most effective for Alex, but every child is different, and like anything else, these oils require experimentation, and treatment with them demands observation.

I find that by tracking my third son's progress and being attentive to the shifts in his energy and activity, I have been able to make changes that support Alex in his journey.

But the decision-making isn't without its difficulties. I noticed not too long ago that Alex was having fewer seizures, but some were very long. This made us decide to add a traditional pharmaceutical, in addition to keeping him on the Charlotte's Web oil.

I don't know what we would do without all the help Paige Figi, the Stanley Brothers, Realm of Caring, Jason Cranford, Haleigh's Hope, our CHOP neurologist, and our team of professional and nonprofessionals has offered and continues to offer. It seems we have acquired a crew. Or, rather, Alex has. Sometimes, I feel as if the rest of us are simply trying to keep up.

My dad always said, "Keep the faith."

Faith, along with our tribe, is what helps us when we hit bumps.

This is a work in progress.

We did need to add Zonisamide in 2017. We were seeing longer seizures. We are still giving Alex oil. In the morning, he'll take CW, and we switched back to evening CW instead of HH. Realm of

---

[2] "CBD is cannabidiol, a major non-psychoactive constituent of cannabis which has multiple pharmacological actions including antioxidant, neuroprotective, anxiolytic, antipsychotic, antiemetic, and anti-inflammatory properties." (Realm of Caring)

Caring was helpful again. Dylan, a staff member at Realm of Caring in Colorado, explained that some children are sensitive to THC. Alex may be one of those. I hadn't realized, until Dylan from ROC enlightened me, that taking Zonisamide with the oil could cause more convulsions. I looked back through my notebooks and realized that there might, indeed, be a correlation. These oils are like any pharmaceutical medicine. Everyone's body responds to every drug differently. We continue to give him CW oil, but we dose it about two hours apart from his Zonisamide, since it can interact if given too close together. These details are important, so although I have tried to thoroughly educate myself, I am grateful to the experts for their insights.

Previously, we had a strict diet for Alex. His GI doctor, Dr. Boyde, was concerned that he was not gaining enough weight again. We introduced a more typical diet. He is down in his seizures from nine per month to four, and they are short. He is gaining some weight again to our relief.

Dylan explained that a healthy "veganish" diet could be helpful too. He said digestion can affect seizures. I believe this. Since these realizations, we've been limiting his gluten and working hard to provide whole, nourishing foods, not just for Alex but for the entire family. As mentioned, we were already trying to eat healthily, but the reminders from Dylan and Alex's doctor were a helpful nudge. We should all be eating clean, healthy foods. Having an additional incentive (supporting Alex) is yet another way he has enriched all of our experiences.

My youngest son is a pillar of strength, and I am encouraged by his desire to grow and to live, to be part of life and to defy the expectations of a culture that can sometimes be down on Down syndrome. Recently, Alex tried to stand at a soccer game for his brother, Sam. It was thrilling. Haleigh's Hope, and Charlotte's Web are magical.

I remain hopeful that one day soon we will be free of this new medication, Zonisamide. For now, I have to admit the seizures, when we see them, are shorter. I know with my heart that the CW oil helps Alex with his quality of life. He still smiles and laughs. He is back to eating everything again. His neurologist says that we can stop the Zonisamide when he is seizure-free. I cannot wait. Fortunately, we have not seen many harmful side effects. I'm praying Alex keeps getting better. I'm praying the end of his seizures are near.

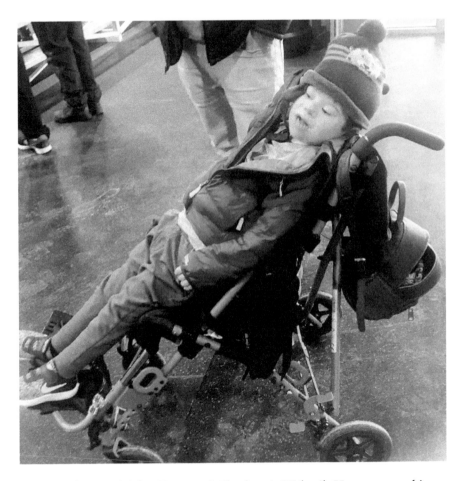

Alex was taking Haleigh's Hope and Charlotte's Web oil. He was not taking any traditional pharmaceuticals here. For the first time ever, Alex tried to stand himself at Sam's soccer game in his wheelchair stroller. This was miraculous.

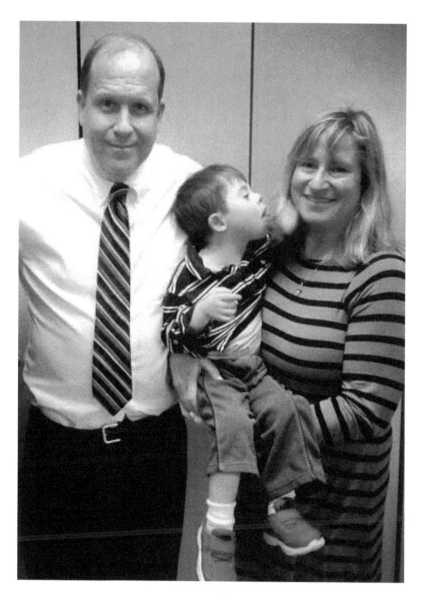

Alex met State Senator Daylin Leach to share his gratitude for Senator Leach's help to legalize medical marijuana in Pennsylvania. Senator Leach courageously fought to help people gain access to medical cannabis in Pennsylvania.

Lessons Alex Taught Me:

- When attempting to solve a difficult problem, especially a medical problem, act like a scientist. Keep track, take notes, ask questions, and listen to the answers.

- Medicine is an art. There is room for grace and inquiry. Don't expect it to be clear cut.

- Science does not always have the answers.

- Physicians do not always know your child best. Even so, finding the right doctor for your family is crucial. The best physicians are the ones who hear you and listen with their hearts.

- While it is always possible to learn from other people's stories, great wisdom and insight comes from trusting one's "Mama gut."

Alex:

It is scary to be asleep and suddenly have no control. My body shakes. I feel like I can't breathe. A storm thunders in my head. It terrifies me. I think that is why I cry so much when it happens. I wish whatever these things were would go away.

6   **Boob**

Getting the note for the six-month surveillance mammogram made me pause. I thought, *I could just ignore it.* My last mammogram, in July, was fine. Why would things change? I had been told I was at a high risk for developing breast cancer, but that was just a warning. Like a yellow light. I could accelerate through it. I didn't have to stop.

In spite of the inner voice urging me to put it off, I went. I did the responsible, adult thing. I always do the responsible, adult thing.

I was working full-time teaching ELL; caring for two dogs, a cat, and a bearded dragon; raising three boys, one who hadn't yet learned to walk or talk; and waking up at night when my youngest's seizures woke me. I had been tired for five years. In addition to all the things on my have-to-do list, my time was occupied trying to stay together, look good, and keep in touch with friends and family.... I didn't have time for any more challenges. Not that life was all a challenge. Quite a lot of it was—is—lovely. And I don't want to give the impression that my entire existence revolves around being a mom. Or a friend. I have my own hobbies, interests, and loves. And I do my best to maintain my marriage.

Michael and I make fancy lunch dates, go to cafes, watch movies, shop, make love, and care deeply about each other. In good times, and challenging times, we stay together. We try to be true to ourselves, which helps us have a better relationship. We have been together for thirty-five years. I met him when I was fifteen and he was eighteen. We know each other well. We feel comfortable together—and connected. We're so connected that I once had a dream about a huge home with rooms everywhere, some with dropcloths covering parts. When I woke up and told Michael about it, he told me he'd had the same dream!

"Let me see this slide." The nurse at the breast center walked me back to the dark room where doctors talked in hushed tones while reading films. My doctor pointed out the tiny white dots on the slide. I looked through my reading glasses at the image of my right boob.

"It looks fine to me."

"Well, I strongly suggest you get a biopsy."

"Why? I did that in 2014. It was fine then, and I think it looks fine now."

As I eyed the films from that day's scan, held side-by-side with the ones from July, a small voice in my head implored me to pay attention to the calcifications. Another, louder, voice screamed, "I can't! I just can't."

Could it be that I'd been given yet another mountain that I would now have to climb? I needed to take care of Alex. I needed to visit my mentally fragile sister. The meds were not helping her schizophrenia, and after seeing my own boys' sibling love, I'd striven to be better to Wendy as an adult than I'd been as a child.

The doctor was gentle but firm. "You need a biopsy," she repeated.

The nurse handed me a paper.

Crying, scared, I drove away.

I phoned my OB/GYN—the same one who had delivered Alex.

Dr. Crate spoke kindly to me, assuring me I could always get a second opinion. I did just that. At 1:00 p.m. the same day.

During my visit to a second doctor at the breast center, I huddled close to another expert as he carefully reviewed the same films as his colleague. "It is true that it does not look hugely different, but I think you should at least get an MRI to be sure."

"No. I had one in 2014. I don't want to go through that again. I really don't think I need one. I'm fine."

The doctor looked at me with understanding in his eyes. "If you choose, you can wait six months, check again, and have the MRI then."

"I choose."

He repeated that I should get the MRI. "Then, at least you will know more."

"Nah, I'll be fine."

He remained unconvinced.

"Can't I just repeat the mammogram in six months?"

The doctor tried, again, to convince me, but I was focused on the tiny sliver of hope.

It does not look hugely different....

I left feeling like I'd made the right decision. I had no time for MRIs, calcified breasts, or cancer scares.

In retrospect, I realize how ridiculous it was for me to think I could sweep my own health needs under the rug. If I was dead, I couldn't help Alex, Josh, or Sam. I thought back to the advice I had received shortly after Alex's birth. The wise words I learned from Joel Osteen's book *Your Best Life Now*, reminding me to practice self-care: "Put your own oxygen mask on first."

No. I can't. My old self-denial mantra was winning again.

As I went through my day, my thoughts kept drifting to my mom. She had just finished her third bout of breast cancer and undergone a double mastectomy, when she phoned me, crying, "I have no boobs anymore."

I told her she just needed to find herself an ass man. Mom exploded in much-needed laughter. She has since recounted this story to everyone, including her mail carrier. I thought of my brave sister-in-law, Ellen. After her double mastectomy, she not only survived, she thrived. She is now happily married, again, and living in a new home in Seattle.

Our family friends, Trish and Rebecca, my mom's college roommate, Barbara Bowman... All these women had gone through cancer. And I knew that if I were to ask them, they'd all tell me that early intervention is essential. Plus, living with Alex was a daily reminder of the importance of trusting both your gut and your doctors. The inner voice warning me not to seek answers wasn't intuition. It was fear.

I texted Ellen: "Hey, freaking out. Had a weird mammogram. One doctor said get a biopsy. One said I could wait six months. All I keep thinking is, if I die...no one will love and help Alex like I do. Anyhow, if you have time, I would love to chat."

Ellen texted back: "Get the biopsy now. Don't freak out. This happened before didn't it? An abnormal mammogram, Call me if you need me."

I explained through yet another text: "It did, which is why I feel like why go through it all again."

Ellen replied: "Better safe than sorry. If G-d forbid it is something, better to catch it early. Gives you more options."

"Thanks, El," I texted back.

Her response: "I'm sorry if I'm not much help. I pretty much sleep-walked through my whole experience. I certainly was not what you would call an educated patient. But I know you shouldn't put off something you can address today, especially when it comes to your health."

Ellen's prompting did the trick. I got the biopsy. When the doctor, the second one that said I could probably wait the six months, phoned me, it was 5:00 p.m. on a Friday.

The boys were running around. Michael was scrambling to get to his racquetball game.

"It is DCIS—*Ductal Carcinoma in Situ.*" The doctor's voice sounded far away on the other end of the line. "A noninvasive cancer."

Cancer.

The word echoed in my head. I repeated it. "Cancer? I thought you were calling to say everything is fine."

I knew Michael could hear me. He left for racquetball anyway. In the movies, when disaster strikes, partners hold each other. But this wasn't the movies. It did, however, conjure memories of a certain set of film. I recalled my numbness and denial when the doctor showed me images of my breasts, dark and slightly fuzzy on the films. Michael reacted as I had at the mammogram. Denial and shock. Michael is the best husband, but we are both chronically afflicted with our own individual to-do lists as well as a litany of family obligations.

I didn't fault Michael for his inability to process my devastating news in the moment. It was Alex's birth all over again. Shock. He needed time to process. Life was not going according to our plan. Michael would eventually comfort and console me. But he needed time. Truth be told, so did I. I was reeling. Luckily, after Michael reset himself, he was my biggest ally and advocate.

After my first surgery, and my second one, he took care of Alex, Josh, and Sam. Caring for Alex is not easy, even when we are both well. If one is down, it is next to impossible. But Michael did it.

After my first surgery, he helped me when I was sick from the anesthesia. I could not move for a week. He brought me Hawaiian Punch. He heated up the mac and cheese my friend, Sara, made me, which, for a long time, was all I was able to eat. As soon as Michael and his racquetball gear were out the door, Josh, then aged fifteen, hugged me. "Mom, I'm sorry. I hope you will be okay."

Fourteen-year-old Sam's face contained no expression, but, the next day, he spent the entire morning with me. He even picked out new Purple Adidas Ultra Boost sneakers for me at the Bryn Mawr Running Company so I could have new sneakers to work out in.

We all show fear and worry in different ways. I learned this from Alex, also known as our "Ups Baby."

The first person to refer to Alex by this nickname was our dear friend and mentor, Tante Jeanette, who went by the name MoonSong. MoonSong has since passed on, but, as a part of her legacy of love, she left Alex a generous monetary gift. Jeanette said Alex would need this. She told me this when she was asking me for our Social Security numbers to arrange for provisions for our youngest child. Her love lives on in our memory of her, as do her everlasting words.

"Our soothing similarities, and our delightful differences are what brings us together," MoonSong said. This is one of her most beautiful quotes. I miss her.

The surgeries were two years ago, in March and April 2017. I had to make plans to take a sabbatical from my work. On my last day of work, before my restoration of health sabbatical, my ELL student, a recent arrival from the Congo, sought me out. With huge eyes, she said, "You are sick, but you will be okay."

She was five. Her name was Faith. I had not said a word to her about the breast cancer. She could not possibly have known. And, yet, like Alex, she had a wisdom that went beyond anything she was able to articulate.

After my second surgery to make sure the stage-one cells found on my stage zero lumpectomy were clear, and a sample of my lymph nodes was taken to make sure they too were clear, I worked hard on visualization. My sister, Susie, had advised me to use visualization as a healing technique. She told me that how a person sees things in their mind can affect the outcome they experience in their life. Just as an athlete sees themselves making the dive, spinning on ice, or executing the jump, I pictured my surgeon, Rick Bleicher, smiling at the post-operation appointment. I imagined him telling me I would be okay.

Each time my thoughts veered to worry and dread, I filled my mind with positive, life-affirming images, and the net result was my positive projections nullified the negative.

My friend, Bina M. Patel, told me the mind is powerful. "Mindfulness works," she explained. "Work at staying strong and keeping your mind in a positive place. Imagine something that gives you joy, or visualize a beautiful place."

As mentioned, Sara would make mac and cheese. I was in love with her mac and cheese. It was the only thing I could eat after the first surgery. The recipe was from Ina Garten, the *Barefoot Contessa*, Sara informed me.

Rebecca Snyder advised that I work out as much as I could so I could let off steam and keep my body strong. These pieces of advice from my sister Susie, Ellen, Bina, Barbara, Rebecca, and other friends worked.

Aunt Paula is my mom's sister in Cincinnati, Ohio. The year I was diagnosed with breast cancer, she learned that my salary would be cut in half. Aunt Paula generously gifted us financially to make up the deficit so our family could focus our energy on getting me well. This kind of sacrifice and kindness is all I hope for my children to learn. What a blessing to have an aunt who sees her family with her heart.

At my post-op visit after the second surgery, Rick opened the door and said, "ALL NEGATIVE."

At first, his doctor-speak was foreign.

Negative...

My heart sank.

Then, I took in his smile and his tone. I grasped his meaning. Negative was a good thing. I hugged him so hard I thought I might hurt him. The relief was strong. Overpowering. I felt myself breathe for what felt like the first time in a long time. Everything suddenly struck me as beautiful. My husband sitting in the chair beside me, the amazing surgeon who I'd come to think of as a friend, the people in the waiting room, even the administrators in charge of scheduling. All my doubts and concerns evaporated.

It's been eighteen months. This energy has stayed with me. I feel young. I want to hike mountains, play my cello, dance in a ballet company, reconnect with people I knew before the diagnosis, and make my home more beautiful. I want to love my family as I've never loved them before. I recall feeling this way in college. A sense of hope washed through me. I don't know why, but this mental image of Banana Republic rhinoceros T-shirts and a sense of wonder enveloped me. Red cowboy boots I had bought in New York City when my sister was at Stern College, a top bright yellow with white lace, and butterfly sleeves I had from childhood, a lavender dress with a pocket full of chewed gum.... It all became clearly focused, like the lens on an expensive camera. My world. My life. My past. The miracle of the present moment.

Anything seems possible now. I am happy. I am strong. I am positive.

I feel like a teenager. Every day strikes me as a gift. I want to unwrap each one and rejoice in all that it contains.

Rick posted something on Facebook that I saw recently, and it really resonates with me. "99.99% of the things we worry about NEVER occur. Consider that the next time you worry."

It has been a full year. I remain up, not down. Blessed. I just had another mammogram, and everything was clear. Even a previously questionable tumor area on my left side disappeared.

Rick said, "Keep doing what you are doing."

In the aftermath of my surgeries, I left a job that was full-time. I work part-time now. I eat as healthily as I can. I limit my alcohol intake. I take CW oil. I drink green tea daily. I do still eat chocolate, but, oh well. I figure life should be enjoyable. I try to stay calm. I watched all the Chris Beat Cancer Square One videos. When he was diagnosed with cancer, Chris did not get the recommended chemotherapy. Instead, he changed his lifestyle, stress level, emotional health, and nutrition. Inspiring! He has since launched books, videos, and websites about his approach. I cannot do all he suggests, but I try to do a lot. And to have fun in the process.

During what I jokingly refer to as "this boob chapter" of my life, I could not hold or care for Alex as I hoped. That was probably the hardest part of it all, and it drove home the need to get assistance. We are still trying to obtain at-home nurse support for Alex. It has been two years without success. There remains a national shortage. Our lawyer at Disability Rights Pennsylvania is trying to help. In the meantime, I do my best to take care of Alex while also taking care of myself.

Lessons Alex Taught Me:

- Medical challenges can become opportunities to tap into the strength of your mind.

- Visualization works.

- Stay positive, even in the midst of adversity.

- Nutrition matters. Eat a healthy diet with moderation as your guide.

- Get a tribe and lean on them when you need them.

- Second and third opinions help.

- Be present.

- Don't think you can do everything alone. Ask for help. Loved ones want to be there for you.

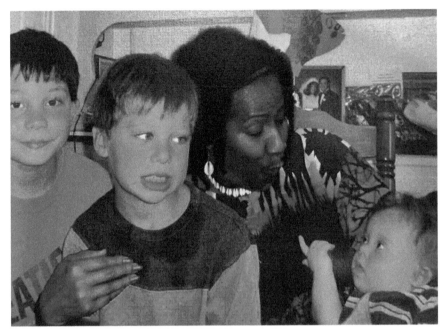

Josh, Sam, and Alex hang out with MoonSong at our home. You can see here how Alex was trying to get MoonSong to think of him as her favorite.

Alex:

Why can't Mom pick me up? Why is she so tired? Why is everyone on edge? Why are my brothers upset? Why is there yelling? My parents look scared.

7 Up Bow, Down Bow

The form came home with a question: *Which instrument would you like your child to learn?* Alex does not walk—yet. Or talk—yet. He finds it challenging to hold a pencil.

Josh played the cello. I played, and still sometimes play, the cello. I wished Alex could play the cello. I filled in the box marked *cello*.

Another form showed up the next day. It instructed me to rent a quarter size cello.

Really?

I rushed to the Music and Arts store in Wayne, Pennsylvania.

"I need a quarter size cello, a bow, some rosin, and *Suzuki Book One*," I told the young man behind the counter.

He wrote *Alex* in big black letters on a tag and attached the tag to the soft instrument case. I thought about the letters we'd hung on my second and third son's door and smiled at the inner acknowledgment of how our lives with Alex have far exceeded our expectations. Alex has exceeded our expectations. But as I left the music store, clutching Alex's instrument to me, I was far from confident.

And yet...

The picture on the next page shows Alex taking his first lesson with his cello teacher, April Beard. The joy, the wonder, and love are seen in his expression. April is the embodiment of all I had hoped for.

She sends me multi-paragraph emails about pizzicato, piano plucking with a soft dynamic level, bow holding, CelloPhant vs. no tool, Alex's attention span, percussion on the cello, music, and more. To get emails like this about our youngest son fills me with a joy that cannot be put into words. Alex is just another fourth grader learning the cello. Each week, after receiving April's email, it takes me a day to respond. I remain that blown away, my doubts eviscerated by awe and gratitude.

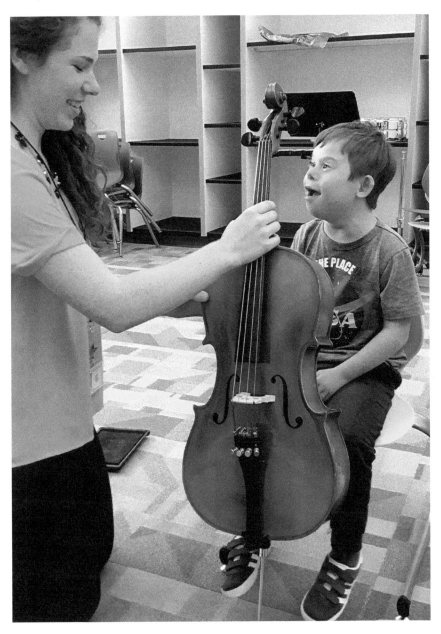

This is the day of Alex's first cello lesson with his cello teacher, April Beard. You can see the joy on his face. It is extraordinary to me that the cello lessons happened at the end of the day, and Alex did not cry or complain he was tired. The thirty-two cello lessons he has had with April Beard are another heart gift that gives me hope. Alex will continue his cello study with April next year at the middle-school level.

April is a gifted teacher. She perfectly balances how to challenge Alex yet meet him where he needs support. She turns the instrument toward him so he can see and hear. He can play percussion on it or do bouncy bowing. April accepts the level of learning within Alex's current reach. She makes educating him look easy. As a result, Alex is learning. He is also cultivating a love for music. I see this experience as setting the stage for our youngest son to touch the stars. And I marvel at what a miracle he is.

As if the photos weren't enough, April started sending videos. Each YouTube video she sends gives us all hope and joy. Alex is fifteen weeks into his lessons now, and as I watch him, courtesy of these captured moments, I can see his progress, not just as a person but as a performer.

Alex has learned a ton about notes and many ways to play the cello. He has experienced having a cellist who travels to China for her music focusing on his learning the instrument. He struggles to hold the bow, and yet is learning to. He is succeeding in ways I never dreamt possible.

His cello teacher isn't simply teaching him how to play. She is helping him understand that he can do things he never imagined possible. He *can* learn. This teacher's teaching has been magic. It has illuminated the intelligence I have always known Alex possesses.

I watch, enthralled, as April issues an instruction and my youngest son takes his entire body and lifts it up higher to show he understands. An *A* string sounds higher than a *D* string. A friend, Brenda Dixon-Gottschild, noted this. Alex's experiences in the music room have translated into other areas of his life. He has started holding objects more at home. He looks at me with a newfound confidence and poise. It is as if, when he sees me seeing him, we both recognize that something has changed. He has an increased awareness. His sense of self and purpose has grown.

Every time I watch my youngest son play, my mind wanders through a maze of memories and I find myself tearing up at the beauty and brilliance of my youngest boy.

His pincer grasp is better since starting the cello, and his grasp on life itself seems to have strengthened. What a gift these cello lessons have been. Alex fills our life with daily music simply by existing, and seeing him respond to the notes and chords of his newfound learning fills us all with a desire to sing.

Lessons Alex Taught Me:

- You can do anything you want.

- Extraordinary teachers are everywhere.

- Learning is easy when you apply yourself, and are willing to try new ways of understanding.

- Music is magic.

- Just because something seems impossible, it may not be.

Alex:

Me? I get to play this beautiful cello? You think I can do it? You believe in me? I get a chance to show what I can learn? Thank you. I am amazing. I won't let you down. Watch what I can do. Look, Mom; I will make you proud.

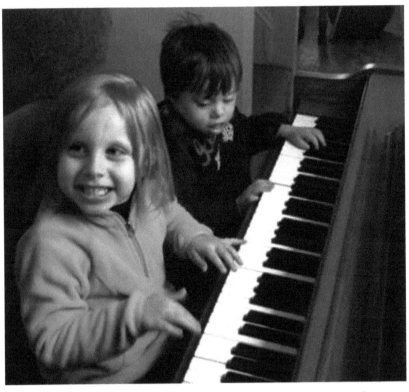

Alex playing the piano with his first friend, Fiona. They met at age four months, and are still friends at age eleven."

8 Architect

When I first set out to write this book, I thought about titling it *Up, Not Down: The Architect of My Soul.* I have since changed the title, but the sentiment remains the same.

Architect: A person who designs buildings and supervises their construction.

Soul: The spiritual, immortal part of an animal or human being.

Alex has rebuilt my soul. The lessons he has brought to my life are too numerous to enumerate, and yet this book is my humble attempt to explain the unexplainable joys of raising a child with Down syndrome.

I hope my story helps you understand what life is like for people who may not be able to express themselves the same as everyone else, but who feel deeply and love deeply, and who are hungry to be treated with kindness and respect.

Trisomy 21 (Down syndrome) symptoms exist along a spectrum. Children and adults with this diagnosis have various complications. Some have serious medical challenges, others learning differences. A range of cognitive and physical effects accompany a Down syndrome diagnosis.

Alex cannot walk or stand on his own yet. He has never crawled. He has trouble moving his body to flip over. He cannot feed or dress himself. He cannot use the facilities, bathe, or brush his teeth alone. Yet.

Every bite and sip of food or drink needs assistance. Every moment he is awake, he needs a helper. When he sleeps, he is monitored on a video baby monitor. The monitor alerts us if his breathing changes, or if he is having a seizure. Whenever it beeps, we rush to him, turn him to his side to breathe, and assess whether or not we need to call 911. If a seizure lasts for more than five minutes, emergency medicine is recommended.

But these are only some of the things about Alex's life. There is so much more to his existence than limitations.

When Alex was three, I ordered an Upsee. An Upsee is a tool that allows a child to walk attached to an adult. Later, I saw a mom, Heather Clark Harris, on Facebook use the Upsee with her son, Clark, in Canada. Clark laughed as his sister kicked the ball to him. I showed the video of Clark kicking the ball and laughing with his sister to Josh and Sam.

Josh was the first to put it on, and Sam kicked a soccer ball to Alex, who immediately let out a sound I had not heard before. My youngest son belly-laughed, hard. Alex loved being in the device. He loves—loves—his big brothers. It cracked him up when Josh or Sam bounced the soccer ball off their heads. I am forever grateful to Clark and his mama for teaching us to inspire Alex's laugh.

All these memories and more have created a tapestry of affection that blankets our family of five. But it also spreads out to cover a larger radius.

As high school students, Josh and Sam each volunteered to help children who had special needs play sports. They have an unshakeable faith in the strength of everyone, including their baby brother.

Josh sees what can be, not just what is. While our family was staying at my mother-in-law's for two months while our home was renovated to accommodate the needs of living with a challenged child and the growing demands of everyone in our family, Josh saw I was about to feed Alex a pesto ravioli and said, "Stop, Mom. Let him do it."

At first, I was annoyed that he corrected me in front of his Grandma Sandy, but I knew he was right. I let Alex hold the fork. Slowly, he brought it to his lips, its prongs spearing the pesto ravioli. I held my breath and then...surprise! He did it!

We were all amazed.

Well, all of us except Josh. Someone snapped a photo.

Alex has mastered playing the cello his way. He has mastered actively listening when someone else is reading aloud. He has mastered making friends and keeping them. He has mastered loving his family. He has mastered eating and drinking. He has mastered using the toilet when given the chance to go on a routine schedule. He has mastered watching movies and shows on Netflix. He has mastered dancing and singing in his own way.

He has become well-known in his community.

He brings light into our world.

Alex plays games in school and goes to recess. He is part of their community of play.

Carrying Alex in and out of our home is not an easy task. We carry him down a path from the car into our home. If we are taking him out, we need to carry him from where we park the car to his stroller.

It wasn't until I began navigating the world with a challenged child that I realized ours is a stair-filled world. (And, I regret to say, a stare-filled world. People can be unfairly judgmental). Sometimes, our family cannot go into a place because it is not wheelchair accessible. We get tired at times from the energy it takes to bring Alex places. While we would not have it any other way, physically it is a challenge for us.

Luckily, however, home has become our sanctuary. Thanks to our wonderful realtor, Tom Lowy, for helping us find our builder. We are grateful to our builder, Brian Borden, owner of BUILT construction. Brian's work has changed our lives and brought peace to our hearts.

My mother-in-law, Sandy Schwartz, and her fiancé, Allen Liss, helped us make our home accessible for everybody. They are two of the kindest, most loving, and positive people I have ever known. Before the renovation, we had to carry Alex up and down extremely steep steps to the one bathroom and his bedroom. If others were using the facilities, it was not fun. Sharing a bedroom with his brother was hard because of seizures.

Each epileptic episode would wake Sam, and as a teen, he did not have privacy. The roof leaked. The floors had holes, and the paint was dark and peeling everywhere. The bathroom had mildew that would not go away. The windows were potential guillotines, which had to be opened and closed carefully. One had a giant hole in it. Our family cat used the hole as his own personal entrance and exit. It was also freezing in the winter and hot in the summer. We did not have heat in our room, and there was no central air conditioner.

With the renovation, the roof was repaired. No more indoor rainstorms in our bedroom. The living room was divided in half. Part is now Alex's room, including a full bathroom of his own. Sam has own room, although he still naps in the living room next to Alex's, and he still likes to study alongside his younger brother.

I think he derives peace from Alex. We all do.

This renovation has made our lives easier with Alex, Josh, and Sam. We are lucky. What a blessing to have a mother-in-law, and a step-fiancé-in-law, who were willing to help.

Recently, Michael left his job. This was an incredible, courageous leap of faith. He is looking for a new path. We are excited to see where he will go next, and what remains in store for our family.

In the past, if my husband had left his job without another, I would have panicked. Now I feel only a deep calm and a hope for the future. I am happy he is doing what makes his heart happy.

I have changed from having Alex in my life. I was always anxious about everything. I am calmer now. I see the big picture. Alex has changed my internal architecture. I see the potential in people. Every day I wake up feels like a present.

My mom's optimism has officially rubbed off on me. I am hopeful for the future.

As I was putting the finishing touches on this book and reflecting upon the ways Alex has helped me evolve and grow, both as a person and a parent, I realized that to keep this story purely in my own, limited viewpoint wouldn't do it justice.

Alex has expanded the minds and hearts of so many. His impact has touched family, friends, teachers, medical professionals, and even strangers on the street. The ripple effect he has had will forever remain unknowable.

My ocean wave son has been touching us all with his healing waters, eroding shores of intolerance and segregation, wearing away at sharpness to create beautiful, multi-colored sea glass. He is everything I never would have asked for yet desperately needed, and, because I am told the same almost daily by others, I decided to ask a select group of family and friends to provide me with a few of the lessons Alex has taught them.

This is by no means a comprehensive accounting. The influx of responses was too overwhelming. Plus, there were a lot of redundancies. Overlapping insights. People expressing the same sentiments in their own, unique ways. But here is a small sample of what people had to say:

- Everyone has a place and purpose in the world. We are expected to be our best. While Alex isn't able to be his best, he has a unique ability to bring out the best in others, especially his parents and brothers. As we move through life, we have certain expectations of how things should be, and sometimes, it's easier to take a lot for granted. Sometimes, we look so far ahead that we forget to appreciate what is really important right now. Thinking about Alex regrounds us. Life doesn't treat everyone fair, and with Alex's needs and personal medical issues, Nancy and Michael have their share of hardships. These things haven't taken them down but made them stronger. We all need to be transformative when things don't go as planned and find a way to continually remake a new normal for ourselves. Not being there all the time, we can't really understand all the daily ups and downs that Nancy and Michael have. But since it involves our family, it's given us deep-set and long-term empathy and compassion. Seeing how Nancy and Michael have arranged to have Alex spend time in public school with his peers makes me think we shouldn't give in too quickly to adapt to what the world expects; sometimes, we need to be advocates and work hard to make the world accept our needs. (**Glenn and Sheryl Schwartz, Alex's aunt and uncle**)

- Nothing is impossible, even when faced with the most daunting of obstacles. Support and love from others can help us succeed. Overcoming obstacles makes success that much more special. No goal is too small, and every victory is worth celebrating! Don't rush the process—everything that is supposed to happen will happen when it is supposed to happen. Alex's inspiration helps me always! ☺ (**Heather, Alex's cousin**)

- The care and love the family gives to Alex every day is wonderful to see, and it has opened my heart to this truly wonderful young child. In spite of his challenges, Alex tries to be part of what is happening around him. This effort on Alex's part is truly inspirational. It reinforces for me that it is possible to conquer every challenge. I always look forward to spending time with Alex and the family. (**Allen Liss, Alex's Grandma Sandy's fiancé**)

- We all face many challenges in our lives, but I learned from my grandson, Alex, that if you try hard enough, you can keep reaching new heights. Most of all, Alex has given me the inspiration to be patient, compassionate, and to always treat everyone with kindness and love. I love you, Alex, and I am so glad that you are part of our family. Hugs and kisses, GaGa Sandy (**Sandy Schwartz, Alex's Grandma "GaGa"**)

- I learned that no matter who you are, when you set your mind to something you are capable of anything! (**Jordan Schwartz, Alex's cousin**)

- I learned what a kind incredible sister, brother-in-law, and nephews I am blessed with. They have superhuman patience and boundless love to give. I learned each person will grow and develop at his or her own pace because each person is a unique soul and gift from above. I learned that each day is a gift, and each new step or milestone is a miracle. I learned to be grateful for all the gifts I was given. I learned that one little boy with his own unique gifts, and challenges can bring so much love and joy into a family and into the world. I learned that everyone has a voice and talents. (**Susie Garber, Alex's aunt**)

- I learned to always try hard, even if it seems impossible. I learned to always smile. I learned to help other people feel happy. (**Elisheva Trachtenberg, Alex's cousin**)

- Where there is a will, there is definitely a way, conventional or unconventional. Everything is better with a team— especially when Alex is on it! Patience leads to endurance and competence. Life is better with extra snacks! (**Katherine Alexander, Alex's occupational therapist**)

- We all can learn so much from Alex, especially not to take life for granted, and to live life to the fullest. (**Kim Gambone, Alex's special education teacher**)

- I think something I've learned is that being different is an opportunity, and it's no fun being vanilla! (**Jake Schwartz, Alex's cousin**)

- Alex has taught me to accept people for who they are, and to appreciate how lucky we all are. (**Sam Schwartz, Alex's brother**)

- I have learned patience, acceptance, love, willpower, and motivation. (**Josh Schwartz, Alex's brother**)

- I've learned never to underestimate someone's abilities, always to inspire others, to be kind, and to be content. Alex has showed me that a simple smile goes a long way, that laughter really is the best medicine, and that it's okay to be cranky. And Alex's relationship with his mother, Nancy, has taught me that a mother's love can give a son an extremely strong voice. (**Michael Schwartz, Alex's father**)

- I have witnessed such love between you and him. There is not anything you would not do for your son. It is inspiring to see such devotion and strength in the daily activities all of you do. It does not seem to faze you one bit; that is what love is.... Alex is so special and a true blessing. I feel very fortunate to have been able to care for him and get to know you over the last three years. (**Barbara Dale, Alex's school nurse**)

- Alex has taught me that every moment we have on this earth is a gift. It is not uncommon to find ourselves wishing time away, calling on more enjoyable times like a vacation or the weekend. We can get so caught up that we forget about the precious moment we are presently in—the only moment that is promised to us. Alex has taught me the importance of slowing down and cherishing every moment I am blessed with in this life. Alex has shown me that no milestone is too small or insignificant. By watching him get stronger and develop new skills over the years, Alex has taught me the importance of celebrating every single accomplishment in life. Most of all, Alex has taught me to show daily gratitude. We too often lose sight of all the great things we have, and the amazing things we are capable of. It seems more natural to compare ourselves to others whom we think are superior in these aspects. I have learned from Alex that we have everything to be grateful for. Every day, every breath, and every ability should give us reason to smile and say "Thank you" for all he has taught me and continues to teach me every day. I am a better person by having this young man in my life. For this reason, and many, many more, I am most grateful for Alex. (**Kristen Culligan, Alex's PCA, personal care assistant**)

Alex:

I feel so special and blessed. I absolutely love my family. My parents and brothers take such good care of me. My parents worry about me all of the time. I wish they could stop worrying. They do so much for me. They prepare unique foods and work at giving me the best medicine. They get up at night when I have a seizure or cry. Ew, I hate those seizures. I hope I don't get them anymore. My parents carry me around everywhere and tell me how they love me so much. When my mom carries me outside and we hear the birds, she tells me, 'The birdies love you; they are saying how cute and smart you are."

Mom takes me to many fun places where we share books, enjoy gardens, and eat delicious treats. Mom hugs me and tells me how amazing I am each day and how I will never know how much she loves me. I love being with my mom and how her perfume reminds me of flowers.

My dad snuggles and swims with me. I love swimming with him. Dad makes the best meals; he is a master chef in the kitchen.

I love my brothers. They are so kind. They play with me and read with me. I love playing soccer with them. Sometimes they watch movies with me.

I love my dogs. I always drop some of my dinner to them. I love my cat. He sleeps next to me in case I have a seizure. He tries to keep me calm. I love my bearded dragon, except when he eats crickets—yuck!

I love the school I go to. My teachers and friends are the best. I love the world. I am so grateful to be in this world with my family.

Mom and Dad, even though, I may not make a Mother's or Father's Day card, or tell you how much I love you, I hope you know I do. I hope you know I think you are the best mom and dad in the whole wide world.

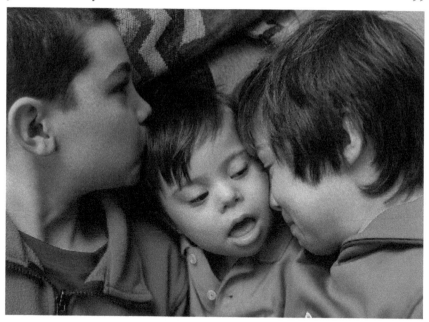

Josh, Alex, and Sam. They share a strong brother love bond.

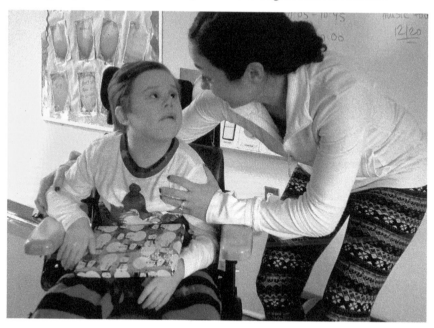

Mrs. Kim Gambone and Alex. Kim Gambone is one the most gifted educators I have ever known. Kim's communication with me every day through written reports complete with smile and frown emojis, daily emails, many phone calls, and conferences instilled confidence that Alex was learning and thriving.

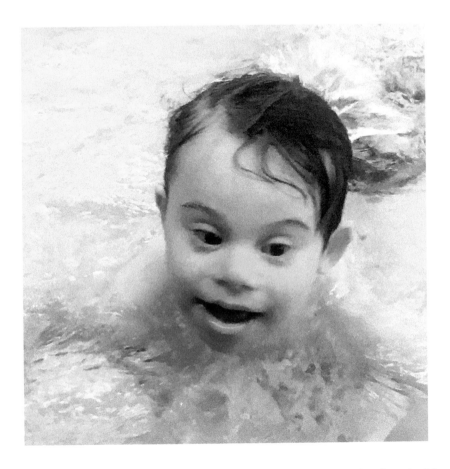

Alex in his happy place. Alex loves to swim. The exercise he does in his swim lessons, and recreational swimming help to keep his seizure count low. The pool is a place where gravity, barriers, and steps do not exist. You can see how blissful Alex is here.

Bibliography

Albom, M. (2002) *Tuesdays with Morrie*. Portland, OR: Broadway Books.

Agus, D. B. (2012) *The End of Illness*. New York: Free Press.

Agus, D. B. (2014) *A Short Guide to a Long Life*. New York: Simon & Schuster.

Agus, D. B. (2016) *The Lucky Years: How to Thrive in the Brave New World*. New York: Simon & Schuster.

Bomer, R.y. (1995) *Time for Meaning: Crafting Literate Lives in Middle and High School*. Portsmouth, NH: Heinemann.

Bomer, R. & Bomer, K. (2001) *For a Better World: Reading and Writing for Social Action*. Portsmouth, NH: Heinemann.

Bowman, B. T. (2002) *Love to Read: Essays in Developing and Enhancing Early Literacy Skills of African American Children*. Silver Spring, MD. National Black Child Development Institute.

Breathnach, S. B. (1995) *Simple Abundance*. New York City: Warner Books.

Breathnach, S. B (1996) *The Simple Abundance Journal of Gratitude*. New York City: Warner Books.

Brecher, Chad. (2017) *The Lost Book of Wonders: A Novel*. Athens, GA: Deeds Publishing.

Byala, S. (2013) *A Place That Matters Yet: John Gubbins's Museum Africa in the Postcolonial World*. Chicago, IL: U of Chicago P.

Calkins, L. (2000) *The Art of Teaching Reading*. London, Gr. Brit.: Pearson.

Calkins, L. (1994) *The Art of Teaching Writing*. Portsmouth, NH: Heinemann.

Calkins, L. (1998) *Raising Lifelong Learners: A Family's Guide*. Da Capo Lifelong Books.

Canfield, J. et al. (1997) *Chicken Soup for the Mother's Soul: 101 Stories to Open the Hearts and Rekindle the Spirits of Mothers*. Deerfield Beach, FL: HCI.

Chödrön, P. (2004) *The Pema Chödrön Audio Collection: Pure Meditation, Good Medicine, From Fear to Fearlessness.* Louisville CO: Sounds True.

Coates, T.. (2015) *Between the World and Me.* New York: Spiegel & Grau.

Coelho, P. (1993) *The Alchemist.* San Francisco, CA: HarperOne.

Copeland, M. (2017) *Ballerina Body: Dancing and Eating Your Way to a Lighter, Stronger, and More Graceful You.* New York: Grand Central Life & Style.

Couros, G. (2015) *The Innovator's Mindset: Empower Learning, Unleash Talent, and Lead a Culture of Creativity.* New York: Dave Burgess Consulting, Inc.

Covey, S. R. (1989) *The 7 Habits of Highly Effective People: Powerful Lessons in Personal Change.* New York: Free Press.

Daniels, E. (2017) *Cooking with Leo: An Allergen-Free Autism Family Cookbook.* New York: Skyhorse.

Dixon-Gottschild, B. (1998) *Digging the Africanist Presence in American Performance Dance and Other Contexts.* New York: Praeger.

Dixon-Gottschild, B. (2005) *The Black Dancing Body: A Geography from Coon to Cool.* London, Gr. Brit.: Palgrave Macmillan.

Dixon-Gottschild, B. (2002) *Waltzing in the Dark: African American Vaudeville and Race Politics in the Swing Era.* London, Gr. Brit.: Palgrave Macmillan.

Dyer, W. W. (2003) *There's a Spiritual Solution to Every Problem.* Fort Mill, SC: Quill.

Fu, Danling. (2003) *An Island of English: Teaching ESL in Chinatown.* Portsmouth, NH: Heinemann.

Garber, S. (2002) *Memorable Characters...Magnificent Stories: 10 Mini-Lessons on Crafting Lively Characters—the Key to Great Student Story Writing.* Bethesda, MD: Teaching Strategies.

Garber, S. (2008) *Denver Dreams.* Lakewood, NJ: Israel Bookshop Publications.

Garber, S. (2013) *Befriend: A Novel.* Brooklyn, NY: Menucha Pub Inc.

Gottlieb, D. (2006) *Letters to Sam.* New York: Gildan Media Corp.

Hampton, Kelle. (2013) *Bloom.* New York: HarperCollins.

Hanh, Thich Nhat. (1988) *The Heart of Understanding: Commentaries on the Prajnaparamita Heart Sutra*. Berkeley, CA: Parallax Press.

Hay, Louise. (1984) *Heal Your Body*. Carlsbad, CA: Hay House.

Heard, G. (1995) *Writing Toward Home: Tales and Lessons to Find Your Way*. Portsmouth, NH: Heinemann.

Hugo, N. R. (2011) *Seeing Trees: Discover the Extraordinary Secrets of Everyday Trees*. Portland, OR: Timber Press.

Jarrett, V. (2019) *Finding My Voice: My Journey to the West Wing and the Path Forward*. New York: Viking.

Kabat-Zinn, J. (1990) *Full Catastrophe Living: Using the Wisdom of Your Body and Mind to Face Stress, Pain, and Illness*. New York: Bantam.

Kohn, L. (2018) *to the moon and back: a childhood under the influence*. New York: Heliotrope Books.

Lama, Dalai. (2009) *The Art of Happiness*. New York: Riverhead Books.

Lynard, K. (2007) *Gifts: Mothers Reflect on How Children with Down Syndrome Enrich Their Lives*. Bethesda: Woodbine House.

Minor, C. (2018) *We Got This: Equity, Access, and the Quest to Be Who Our Students Need Us to Be*. Portsmouth, NH: Heinemann.

Morton, H. C. (1995) *The Story of Webster's Third: Philip Gove's Controversial Dictionary and Its Critics*. Cambridge, Gr. Brit.: Cambridge UP.

Noah, T. (2016) *Born a Crime*. New York City: Spiegel & Grau.

Obama, B. (2004) *Dreams from My Father: A Story of Race and Inheritance*. New York: Broadway Books.

Obama, M. (2018). *Becoming*. New York: Crown.

O'Reilley, M. R. (1998) *Radical Presence: Teaching as Contemplative Practice*. Portsmouth, NH: Boynton/Cook Publishers Heinemann.

Osteen, J. (2004) *Your Best Life Now*. Winnipeg, Canada: Word Alive.

Phillips, S. (October 20, 2016) BBC Documentary. *A World Without Down Syndrome*. You Tube. https://m.youtube.com/watch?v=F-SSIwVZeWs

Pliskin, Zelig. (1983) *Gateway to Happiness*. Jerusalem, Israel: Aish Ha Torah Publications.

Polacco, P. (2010) *The Junkyard Wonders*. New York City: Philomel Books.

Prager, D. (1998) *Happiness Is a Serious Problem: A Human Nature Repair Manual*. New York: William Morrow.

Ruiz, D. M. (1997) *The Four Agreements*. San Rafael, CA: Amber-Allen Publishing.

Silver, G. (2009) *Anh's Anger*. Berkeley, CA: Plum Blossom.

St. James, E. (1995) *Inner Simplicity: 100 Ways to Regain Peace and Nourish Your Soul*. New York City: Hyperion.

Strahan, Ml. (2015) *Wake Up Happy: The Dream Big, Win Big Guide to Transforming Your Life*. Australia: Atria/37 INK.

Stevenson, B. (2015) *Just Mercy: A Story of Justice and Redemption*. New York City: Spiegel & Grau.

Walsh, R. (2016) *A Parent's Guide to Public Education in the 21st Century: Navigating Education Reform to Get the Best Education for My Child*. New York: Garn Press.

Wiesel, Elie. (1982) *Night*. New York: Bantam Books.

Winfrey, O. (2017) *The Wisdom of Sundays: Life-Changing Insights from Super Soul Conversations*. New York: Flatiron Books.

Wolpe, D. J. (2008) *Why Faith Matters*. San Francisco: HarperOne.

Wolpe, D. J. (1992) *In Speech and In Silence*. New York: Henry Holt & Co.

Websites

www.noahsdad.com (Blog, Rick Smith)

www.charlottesweb.com (Stanley Brothers)

www.floweringhope.co (Jason Cranford)

www.rainbowplantlife.com (Nisha Vora)

www.TheRoc.us (Heather Barnes Jackson)

www.terravidahc.com (Chris Visco)

Acknowledgments

I am grateful to many people for inspiring this book. My boys, Josh, Sam, and Alex amaze me, daily. My husband, Michael Scott Schwartz, offers love, kindness, and laughter and has fathered the three greatest gifts in this life. I am thankful to my mom, JoAnne Liebenberg Levine, for her enthusiasm, love and guidance; her optimism is contagious. I am grateful to my dad, Martin Levine, for his love of literacy, dedication to his three girls, and love of education. I am thankful to my teachers at Teacher College Reading and at the Writing Project, Columbia University for helping me to understand the power of education. I am grateful to my sister, Susie Garber, for reading several drafts of the *Up, Not Down Syndrome* manuscript. It was her idea to add Alex's voice, and I think it helped tremendously.

Although so many of my friends have had a direct impact on my life and work, I feel compelled to mention by name Sara Byala, Chad Brecher, Jane Dugdale, Barbara Bowman, Valerie Jarrett, Brenda Dixon-Gottschild, David Agus, Ginnelle Bespa, Noriko Lovasz and Lisa Kohn. Thank you to Jeanette Mallory-Hill, also known as MoonSong, and Aunt Paula. Thank you to my book group—they feel more like family than friends and they helped make this project a reality.

I am thankful to Sandy Schwartz, Allen Liss, my nieces, nephews, aunts, uncles, cousins, friends, colleagues, students, students' parents, principals, and the Gryphon café. I did most of the writing for this book at the Gryphon café in Wayne, Pennsylvania, fueled by extra hot lavender lattes. I am grateful to Steve and Ramon at FedEx for always helping me get my work where I needed it to go.

Thank you to my breast and best surgeon, Dr. Rick Bleicher. I am grateful to him for saving my life, my boobs, and my marriage (not necessarily in that order).

Thank you to Paige Figi for her ability to share her journey with others and for inspiring me to do the same; to Jason Cranford for all the work he does, and the Stanley Brothers and the Realm of Caring for vastly improving the quality of Alex's life. Thank you to Daylin Leach, Lolly Bentch, and the producers at CNN.

Thank you to Suli Holum for writing *A Fierce Kind of Love*, a play that includes parts of my and Alex's story; to David Bradley for his extraordinary direction of the play, and to Dr. Dan Gottlieb for featuring it on NPR's *Voices in the Family*. Thank you, too, to actor Lee Ann Etzold for her performance of our story and all the actors in the play.

Thank you to Francis Dunnery for his gift of music. His was the soundtrack that accompanied much of my writing. Thank you to Rabbi David Wolpe for always reminding me to keep the faith.

Thank you to the friends Alex has made and their moms, Shannon O'Donnell Grimes and Julie Goldberg Levick—your friendships are extraordinary. I am grateful to Alex's teacher, Mrs. Kim Gambone, and his helper Kristen Culligan. Thank you to April Beard, Alex's cello teacher, for challenging and supporting Alex. The team Alex has for physical therapy, occupational therapy, and speech therapy is wonderful. To Alex's neurologist at Children's Hospital of Philadelphia (CHOP), I thank you for your willingness to explore new ideas.

I am grateful to my developmental editor, Daralyse Lyons, for helping me clarify and focus my message and to my publisher, Victor R. Volkman, at Modern History Press, for believing in the power of our story.

About the Author

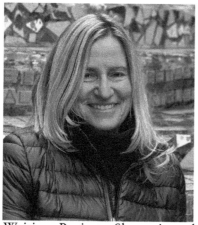

Nancy Schwartz has taught in Pennsylvania for twenty-six years. She holds certificates as an ESL program specialist, reading specialist, and elementary and early education educator. Nancy's undergraduate degree came from Temple University, and she attended graduate school at Saint Joseph's University. Nancy spent several summers studying at the Teachers College Columbia University, Reading and Writing Project. She enjoys ballet, reading, writing, art, fashion, animals, music, and, most of all, motherhood. This is her first book. You can find more photos and stories on her website www.UpNotDownBook.com.

Index

Y

Yoga on Main, 5

Z

Zonisamide, 74, 75

CPSIA information can be obtained
at www.ICGtesting.com
Printed in the USA
BVHW020517120222
628751BV00001B/1

9 781615 994625